THE
GUT HEALTH COOKBOOK

Low-FODMAP Vegetarian Recipes for IBS and Sensitive Stomachs

SOFIA ANTONSSON

Translated by Ellen Hedström

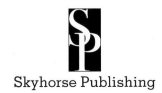

Skyhorse Publishing

Skyhorse Publishing books may be purchased in bulk at special discounts for sales promotion, corporate gifts, fund-raising, or educational purposes. Special editions can also be created to specifications. For details, contact the Special Sales Department, Skyhorse Publishing, 307 West 36th Street, 11th Floor, New York, NY 10018 or info@skyhorsepublishing.com.

Skyhorse® and Skyhorse Publishing® are registered trademarks of Skyhorse Publishing, Inc.®, a Delaware corporation.

Visit our website at www.skyhorsepublishing.com.

10 9 8 7 6 5 4 3 2

Library of Congress Cataloging-in-Publication Data is available on file.

Cover design by Daniel Brount
Cover photo credit: Ulrika Pousette
Interior illustrations by Surabhi Takker

Print ISBN: 978-1-5107-5041-8
Ebook ISBN: 978-1-5107-5043-2

Printed in China

CONTENTS

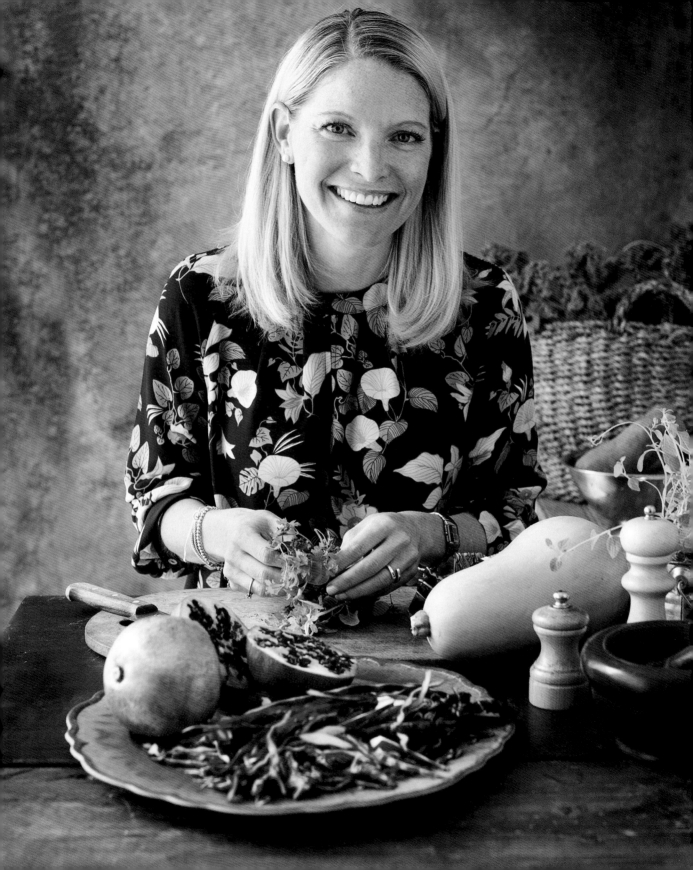

5

You can eat vegetarian, even with a sensitive gut!

I love the gut—there is no more interesting system to study in my opinion. These days I also love my own stomach. I've had IBS since I went to high school, and I know how hard it is to constantly have to think about your gut and make allowances for it. Thanks to FODMAP (which you will shortly find out more about), I no longer need to think about my gut as often. I've also had the opportunity to help thousands of people get "happier" guts just by changing their diets. After writing two cookbooks, a book on bread, and a factual book on the gut, it's finally happened: I get to write a vegetarian cookbook for those who suffer from IBS. Finally anyone with a sensitive gut can eat vegetarian!

Vegetarian food has gone from being synonymous with an alternative lifestyle to being commonplace at the dinner table. More and more of us want to reduce meat consumption, and no one bats an eye if you ask for a vegetarian meal these days. Whether you've just discovered

If you see this sign it means the recipe is vegan

> "We really need to do something to save our planet, and reducing meat consumption is an important but fairly easy solution."

vegetarianism, are an old hand, or just someone who wants to eat less meat, but not go completely vegetarian, this book is for you. Especially if you have a gut that's not quite in balance, which is very common. If you have IBS, a gut that likes to remind you of its presence, or are vegetarian or vegan and hate walking around like a huge gas factory, then carry on reading. The recipes in this book are adapted for a FODMAP diet, which is the most effective method there is to reduce stomach problems.

If you know about the FODMAP diet, you might be thinking, *but how can you combine this with a vegetarian diet?* This is where this book comes into the picture. It will guide those of you who follow a FODMAP diet and at the same time want to reduce meat consumption and eat a more green diet. I'll be holding your hand to make sure it's as easy as possible for you because it shouldn't be more complicated just because you want to eat less meat; that can cause more stress, and, as we know, stress is not good for the gut. I want to make the whole thing much easier, so that those of you with a troublesome gut can make the choice not to eat meat.

This book is also a bit of a personal mission. We really need to do something to save our planet, and reducing meat consumption is an important but fairly easy solution. So if you, like me, want to eat less meat, then let's do this—for your body of course, but especially your gut, as well as the environment, animals, and your wallet.

Sofia Antonsson
Certified Dietician Belly Balance

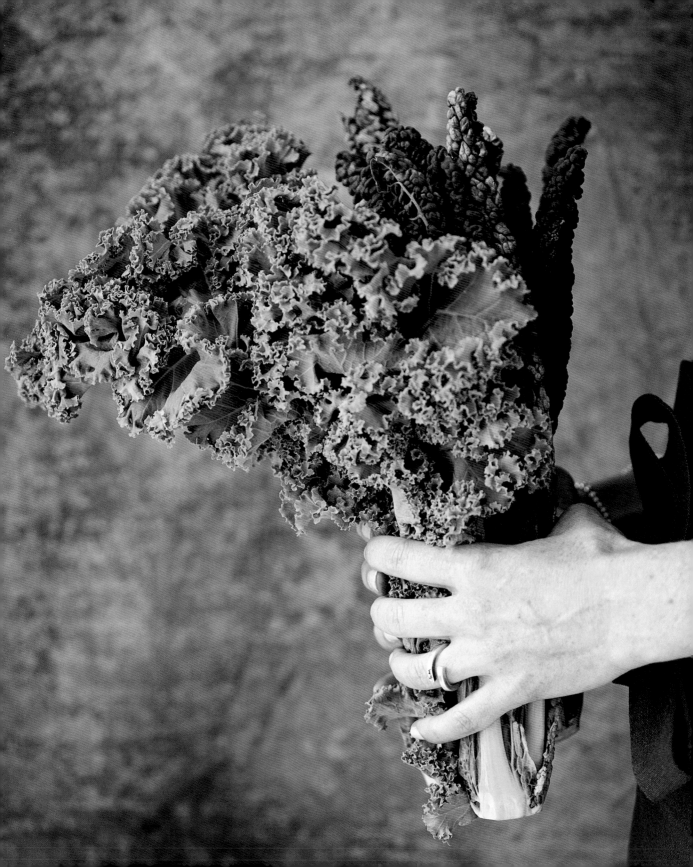

Can you really not eat anything anymore?

Arsenic in your rice, colon cancer from meat, cyanide in flaxseed, flame retardants in salmon, carcinogenics in mushrooms—the list is endless. If you are interested in eating healthily there is a lot to think about. You might be thinking that there is no point in this food stuff and you might as well pop a pill instead.

Food is not the most fantastic thing ever. If we look at it from the point of view that choosing the right food can keep us fit and healthy, then things suddenly seem a bit easier and more fun. In addition, there is constant research telling us that we can influence aging and the risk of illness by the food choices we make.

Despite all the warnings, there is rarely any risk when we eat a normal amount, but as with everything in life, we shouldn't overconsume.

My tip: Eat a normal amount of everything and you will be fine. I'm talking about balance—even if it sounds a bit boring.

YOU ARE WHAT YOU DON'T EAT

The "free from" movement has well and truly taken hold. Fifty percent of Swedes now regularly eat products labeled "free from" such as gluten-free and lactose-free foods, despite only around 1 to 3 percent having celiac disease (gluten intolerance), and around 5 percent being lactose intolerant. There is a bit of a difference between fact and reality, in other words. What is the reason for this? One reason is that food is strongly related to who we are and our identity, and by choosing to eat some foods over others, we reflect who we are. To select some foods over others is also a sort of revolt against the

9

"Learn about
what you can
eat, and choose
to add, rather
than remove,
foods."

establishment, or even the medical profession. Many people think, *if I don't get help I'll find another way or do it myself.* The fact that doctors have gone from being gods to merely being guides is because many people are taking their health in their own hands. Any dietary changes that lead to better health are of course good, but if you have IBS, it is not always best to start meddling with it yourself. The risk is that you remove the wrong things and end up in a circle of constant testing. This causes more stress, which is certainly not going to help your stomach.

My tip: Learn about what you can eat, and choose to add, rather than remove, foods.

FOOD 2.0

We don't just want to eat food because it tastes good anymore; food also needs to give us something. We seem to need even more due to our intensive lifestyle (high tempo, focus on achievement, and so on), which leads to us to needing more nutrients. We feel good if we add some anti-inflammatory turmeric, or eat food that feeds our gut flora, or know the name of the farm that grows our carrots, or what feed the animals have been eating.

But is it really as simple as drinking a shot and then everything is hunky dory? Sadly not. To feel better we need to have a holistic view of how we live. Our lifestyle, especially stress, affects our body negatively and creates inflammations and impair our gut flora. To try and eat clean and unprocessed food as much as possible is a good way to increase nutrients, but we can't compensate for our consumption of soda and candy with a green drink now and again.

My tip: We need to eat more vegetables, fruit, and berries. If we start with this it will be less complicated and overwhelming.

What is IBS?*

IBS (irritable bowel syndrome) is a so-called functional gut disorder. This means there is no evidence of anything being wrong with the gut, it just doesn't work as well as it should. IBS is also known as irritable colon, irritable bowel, spastic bowel, and nervous colon. Between 15 and 20 percent of the world's population suffer from IBS, and 70 percent of those persons are women. Men also get IBS, but don't seek treatment to the same extent.

The number of children and teenagers with gut problems is also increasing, and studies have shown that there is a link to an increase in stress and the pressure to perform. Historically, IBS has been seen as a "vague" diagnosis that can't be treated. These days we know that most people can be helped through dietary changes and through dealing with stress.

You can get IBS at any time of life, even though the usual age of onset for the illness is before thirty to forty years of age. It's not unusual for me to meet persons who have suffered stomach problems for years without getting the right help. I often hear from my patients how their problems started:

- *In infancy:* Maybe you were told your stomach was always bloated or that you were constantly constipated.
- *School age:* Increased stress and pressure, as well as a resistance to go to the toilet in school.
- *After a stomach infection:* The gut never quite recovers after an infection due to an imbalance in the gut flora.
- *After an extended period of stress:* Gut flora is affected by stress, as well as communication from the gut to the brain.

SYMPTOMS OF IBS

Common symptoms
Gas, bloating, pain/discomfort, diarrhea, constipation, irregular bowel movements, incomplete defecation (a feeling that you have not fully emptied your bowels).

Less common symptoms
Nausea, urgent need to urinate, pain in the shoulder area, fatigue, digestive problems (heartburn, nausea, burping).

Cause for concern
Blood in the stool, unintentional weight loss, fever, onset after forty-five years of age. *These symptoms are not related to IBS and should be investigated further!*

IBS can be divided into three diagnostic groups with around 30 percent of people in each group:
IBS-C Constipation predominant: less than three bowel movements a week with hard stools.
IBS-D diarrhea predominant: more than three bowel movements per day with loose or liquid stools.
IBS-M: Mixed constipation and diarrhea.

12

It is not entirely clear why people get IBS, but several factors are known to contribute. We know that a person can have:

- *Stronger or weaker reflexes.* A need to rush to the toilet in the middle of dinner or to never feel the urge to go.
- A *change in gut flora.* This can appear after an infection or course of antibiotics.
- *Low-level inflammation.* A change in communication between gut bacteria, the immune system, and brain.
- *Motility dysfunction.* The intestine works in an on/off position and gases get trapped in the stomach.
- *Increase of nerve endings in the intestine.* More signals than usual go between the gut and the brain, and the gut makes itself more known.

The diagnosis of IBS is often given after tests for celiac (gluten intolerance) and lactose intolerance have been negative. Sometimes an examination of the large intestine is done using a camera (colonoscopy). Occasionally the doctor is unable to give a diagnosis despite investigations and testing, and in these cases the safest way is to try dietary treatment. However if you do want a diagnosis, which you have the right to have, change doctors!

IBS is affected by both diet and stress. For some people 80 percent is about diet and 20 percent about stress, while for others it is the opposite. As changes in diet can give fairly quick results, it's best to start here. Stress levels will automatically reduce, and it should be clearer then what needs to be done.

"IBS is affected by diet and stress. As changes in diet can give fairly quick results, it's best to start here."

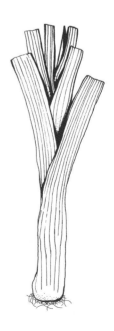

13

What is FODMAP?*

fermentable oligo-, di-, mono-saccharides, and polyols

FODMAP is a dietary treatment and the most effective one we have for IBS. The word FODMAP is an acronym of a group of fermentable carbohydrates (fermentable oligo-, di-, mono-saccharides, and polyols) that are difficult to break down for those who suffer from IBS. So what makes FODMAP so special? Well the method helps 75 percent of all those who suffer from IBS simply by dietary changes and no medication. It is not a fad diet and won't make you thinner, but I can almost promise you that your gut will thank you.

FODMAP CATEGORIES
FODMAP indicates different types of dietary fiber and sugars that people with IBS find difficult to break down and deal with. Instead of being quietly digested and absorbed, they become fast food for our gut bacteria that have a field day in our large intestine. This results in symptoms such as gas, rumbling, and water imbalance; that is, a generally unhappy gut.

FODMAP can be divided into four categories (see next section). Treatment is undertaken in three steps and is based on the traffic light system:
- *Elimination.* Only eat foods marked green.
- *Reintroduction of limited foods.* Add foods marked orange.
- *Reintroduction of forbidden foods.* Add foods marked red.

By first removing foods that we know elicit symptoms in most people, and then reintroducing them in a controlled manner, you can easily see what is causing your stomach problems. You can then control your symptoms by making conscious food choices. If you choose something on the red list, you might have problems, but if you are aware of this, then the symptoms are not as difficult to deal with. The goal with FODMAP is that after six to twelve months you should have identified ten to fifteen foods that you know you should avoid.

FODMAP'S 4 CATEGORIES

1. Fructose

Fruit sugar found in some fruits, vegetables, and honey.

2. Lactose

Sugar found in milk from cows, goats, and sheep.

3. Oligosaccharides

Fiber in cereals, legumes, onion, and garlic, among other things.

4. Sugar alcohols

Sweeteners such as xylitol and sorbitol in chewing gum and throat tablets. They occur naturally in avocado, mushrooms, and cauliflower.

15

THE BUCKET

You can view your stomach as a bucket. When you eat food containing "bad" carbohydrates or FODMAPs, the bucket becomes full because the gut struggles to break them down. When the bucket is full and overflows, you start getting symptoms. By only eating certain foods, you keep the bucket empty, and in this way you create space to eat foods with FODMAPs without getting any symptoms. The bucket empties around once every twenty-four hours depending on the speed of your gut.

WHEN DO SYMPTOMS APPEAR?

Surely, the most natural thing is to see how you feel after you have eaten something? If you don't feel well, then you assume what you ate didn't agree with you. It is not that simple. The food finds its way to the stomach, but it is not until it reaches the large intestine that the IBS symptoms appear. Food that has just been eaten pushes other food through the gastrointestinal tract, so instead you need to consider what you ate at your last meal, or even two meals before that, which has now made its way to the large intestine. It can start to get a bit complicated.

My tip: Keep a food and symptom diary for a few weeks to see what is causing symptoms.

LOW FODMAP IS NOT NO FODMAP

Following the FODMAP diet is a process that takes place over a period of time and happens in several steps. By increasing your intake of foods with FODMAPs, you can understand what your tolerance level is for the different groups, and in this way control your symptoms. At the same time, your gut bacteria get the nutrients they need and your diet doesn't become unnecessarily rigid. Your diet should not consist of FODMAP-free food forever; however a low amount of FODMAPs usually work fine, such as some honey, a bit of avocado, or onion in stock. As long as the total amount is not too high, your bucket will not overflow. When you know what or which categories work better or worse for you, then you can eat foods that contain some FODMAPs. This makes life much easier and you can choose those times that you might want or need to eat more FODMAPs.

HOW TO HAVE A HAPPY GUT

You can try FODMAP whether you have an IBS diagnosis or just have a troublesome stomach. Before you start, it's best to check that you don't have celiac disease (gluten intolerance). After this you can go ahead and begin. At www.bellybalance.se you can go through the program "A balanced gut," which combines FODMAP with stress management. The program helps 85 percent of people and at the same time you get the support from a dietician. If you have had ongoing gut issues always seek advice from a doctor.

GLUTEN OR FODMAP?

Gluten is the protein in wheat, corn, and rye. It can't ferment in the stomach, but it is not the reason for bloating. So, it is easy to assume that this is a case when you eliminate bread and your gut will suddenly be calm. What is going on? Well, when you remove bread and pasta, you remove the gluten, but you also remove the fiber (oligosaccharides, which is a FODMAP), which cause the stomach to bloat and leaves it bubbling and gurgling. Gluten does not give any nutrients to humans, but makes the bread nice and fluffy.

Spelt has a different gluten structure than wheat and is healthier. In addition, spelt doesn't contain as much FODMAPs (oligosaccharides) as wheat. This is why spelt bread is a good alternative for those with IBS and even better if it is baked with sourdough. Both gluten and oligosaccharides are partially broken down when baking with sourdough. What you really want to avoid is pure wheat gluten, which is often added to factory-baked bread to make it fluffy, easy to handle, and quick to rise. This is great for the bakery, but not as good for your gut.

FODMAP + VEGETARIAN FOOD = LOVE!

So how do you eat according to the FODMAP diet if you are a vegetarian or vegan? It can sound complicated at first, but with some planning and knowledge, it is simple, and the recipes in this book provide a great place to start.

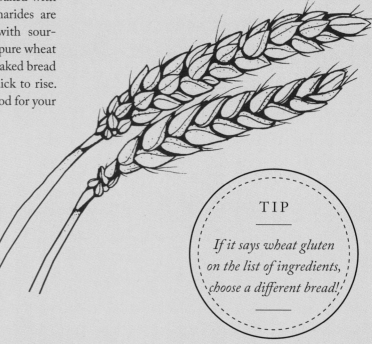

TIP

If it says wheat gluten on the list of ingredients, choose a different bread!

17

Gut flora or gut microbiota

Gut flora is a hot topic right now, as people are starting to understand that the bacteria that live in our gut can affect the manifestation of some of our more common illnesses. Bacteria help us to absorb nutrients from food, but they also communicate with our immune system, endocrine system, and brain. Having a harmonious gut bacteria makes us happy and healthy, but how can you achieve a balanced gut flora? To start, a large part of our gut flora is hereditary on our mother's side. During pregnancy, birth, and breastfeeding, the mother's gut flora is transferred to the infant. The cause of the remainder of our gut flora's actions is a million-dollar question, as no one really knows for sure, even if lots of people think they know. The reason it's a hard nut to crack is:

1. We all have different gut bacteria with a variety of bacterial species and different amounts of bacteria.
2. We don't know what a normal or optimal gut bacteria looks like, as it is unique to every individual.
3. You need a fairly big change in diet over a long period of time before you see changes in gut flora.

This doesn't mean that you can't change your gut flora—of course there are things you can do that are good for the gut without having to turn your life upside down. You might have read about mixing green drinks, eating turmeric, not heating up your food, and avoiding gluten, lactose, and sugar? The question is how many of us have the energy for such extreme diets, not to mention the stress of trying to make daily life function with all these considerations. So instead of going all in and being consumed by a diet for three days before you give up, my advice is to start small and do one thing at a time. We know gut bacteria likes fiber, which we can see when we compare the gut flora in people who eat a diet with a high level of red meat, sugar, and too little fruit and vegetables, as opposed to people with a high intake of plant-based fiber. The diversity of bacterial strains in the gut is larger in those people who eat more fiber. It is also important to avoid things that bacteria dislike. Sugar and red meat are fairly easy to avoid, but the largest threat to our gut bacteria is probably stress. It is worth thinking a bit about this—if you get stressed trying to make a healthy green drink in the morning, then don't do it. The two will cancel each other out.

My tip: Eat fiber and try and avoid stress, even during pregnancy and breastfeeding. Your children will thank you.

GUT FLORA AND FODMAP

Many foods that contain FODMAPs, such as onion, garlic, artichoke, wheat, and rye, are prebiotic. This means that they feed our gut bacteria. Reducing the amount of FODMAPs can also affect the gut flora. The largest effect is during the elimination phase, and it has been shown that the amount of bifidobacteria in the gut reduces during elimination. There are simply not enough food for that genera. The change is not permanent, however, and once you start reintroducing foods, the amount of bacteria will increase again.

My tip: Follow the whole treatment and make sure you reintroduce as many foods as possible to make your bacteria happy.

PREBIOTICS

Prebiotics are food for gut bacteria. Especially good is the prebiotic known as resistant starch. As it is a bit harder for those with IBS to eat varied foods in larger amounts, at least to begin with, you can choose one of the suggestions below and eat them a bit more frequently to ensure you get enough resistant starch.

- *Kiwifruit*
- *Canned lentils*
- *Bananas, green and unripe*
- *White cabbage*
- *Oats*
- *Sourdough bread*
- *Broccoli*
- *Arugula*
- *Cold, boiled potatoes*
- *The green part of scallions and leeks*

PROBIOTICS

You can also take supplement in the shape of a probiotic, which means you get an immediate addition of bacteria. There are two main rules:

1. Always take a supplement with a wide variety of bacterial strains.
2. Always take probiotics with food.

Supplements with lactobacillus and bifidobacterium are especially good during the elimination phase.

19

BRAIN-GUT-GUT-BRAIN

The gut and brain communicate with each other with the help of neurohormones, or neurotransmitters, that gut bacteria produce. Most of the information goes via the vagus nerve from the gut to the brain, but there are even signals from the brain to the gut. If you have IBS, you get more signals from the gut to the brain and therefore sense your gut more than others might. The brain also puts extra focus on the stomach, as there are so many signals coming from the stomach, which creates a vicious circle.

My tip: Try eating according to the FODMAP diet. When the stomach calms down, the signals between the gut and the brain reduce and you will feel less stressed.

STRESS, THE BRAIN, AND THE GUT

Stomach problems cause stress, and stress causes stomach problems, so what came first? The chicken or the egg? Studies show that many of those who seek help for IBS also suffer from mental health problems such as panic disorder and depression. Among women, stomach issues are rife, and many women report that stress, often caused by putting pressure on themselves, is the cause of these stomach issues. There is every possibility that this is the case, as gut bacteria is affected by long-term stress; so it seems obvious that the stomach will start to cause problems after a while. It could also be that the immune system becomes affected, and that you get sick, and in turn need to take antibiotics, which causes even more imbalance in the gut flora.

My tip: Have a think about what is causing you stress, avoid antibiotics, and, if you can, lower your expectations of yourself.

Have a think about what is causing you stress, avoid antibiotics, and, if you can, lower your expectations of yourself.

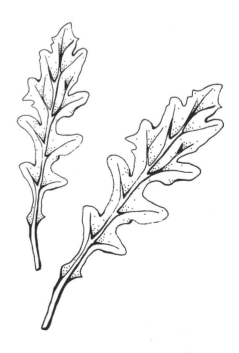

TIPS TO DE-STRESS

Don't get wound up. Consider if it is worth putting pressure on your body before you get angry or irritated.

You're good enough. Stop trying to overachieve. Lower your expectations and see what happens.

Say no. No one will think any worse of you!

Be in your body. Think about what you want, what makes you feel good, and what you enjoy. Not what others say, expect, or think.

Media break. Skip the news, Facebook, and Instagram for a week. If something important happens, you will still find out about it.

Stop multitasking and start mono-tasking. The brain is not designed to do several things at once, we just think it is more effective this way. It rarely, or never, works.

Breathe. Listen to your breath and feel yourself relax. By breathing fewer than eight deep breaths per minute, your parasympathetic nervous system, which is connected to the stomach, is activated.

It sounds like a cliché: "If you stress less your stomach will feel better!" But the fact is that we have to do something concrete to reduce our tempo, reduce the flow of information, and lower the stress levels in our body, otherwise we'll get sick. So take a deep breath, and be inspired by a greener and greater life!

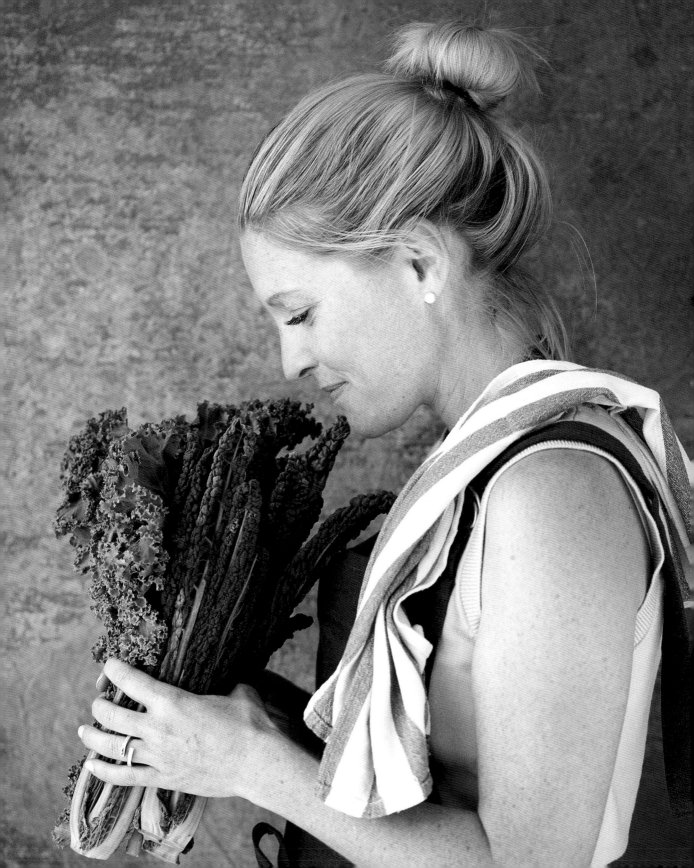

What is vegetarian food?

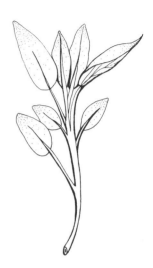

Right, so it is time to talk about what this book is all about: vegetarian food. The term "vegetarian" doesn't mean the samething today that it did twenty years ago, but below are a few definitions of the different terms:

- *Vegetarian or ovo-lacto vegetarian.* A diet with no meat, fish, or chicken but dairy products and eggs are allowed.
- *Vegan.* A diet with no animal products. Hard core, but healthy for us humans.
- *Demi-vegetarian.* Vegetarian food with the addition of chicken, fish, and seafood.
- *Pescatarian.* Vegetarian food with the addition of fish and seafood.
- *Stockholm vegetarian.* A term that seems to mean someone who eats vegetarian when it suits them.
- *Flexitarian.* A new term that means that you try and eat less meat without completely abstaining.

More and more people are choosing to reduce meat consumption and eating more green food.

- *Raw food.* Vegan diet where the food cannot be heated over 107½ degrees as they are thought to lose important nutrients at any higher temperature and at the same time unhealthy substances are produced.
- *Plant-based diet.* It is different from vegetarian and vegan food as the focus is on fruit, vegetables, cereals, nuts, and seeds and the diet avoids meat substitutes and processed foods.
- *Fruitarian.* A diet based wholly on fruit, berries, seeds, and nuts.
- *Climatarian.* The main goal with this diet is to affect the climate as little as possible. That means, apart from eating lots of vegetables, to choose locally produced foods, choose pork and chicken over beef and lamb, and to use all parts of the animal to reduce waste.

23

PLANT-BASED IS THE NEW BLACK

Most people understand that we are what we eat. That is why more people choose to eat vegetarian, not just for ethical reasons, but for our bodies and our health. If you look at the United States, there is a clear trend of an increase in plant-based diets. A vegetarian diet can technically consist of chips and soda, but plant-based means that you are actually eating healthily. More and more studies indicate that a plant-based diet can help reduce the risk of many illnesses such as obesity, high blood pressure, and diabetes.

My tip: Try a plant-based diet and see how your body reacts.

FOR YOUR HEALTH AND BODY

Did you know that 900,000 people in Sweden take antidepressants? Some of those have been given antidepressants because of IBS (which is starting at the wrong end, as most of those with IBS can be helped by changing diet). Most people who use antidepressants, however, are just depressed, and diet and lifestyle are often contributing factors. We know that stress affects us negatively, but some foods are related to inflammation in the body, which in turn increases the risk of depression. White flour, red meat, and sugary drinks are all linked to an increased risk of depression. We feel better and happier if we eat vegetables. When the level of nutrients increase, we get to go to the toilet properly and feel pleasantly satiated.

My tip: Do you have IBS? Change your diet before you start taking medication.

More and more studies indicate that a plant-based diet can help reduce the risk of many illnesses.

IS MEAT AS DANGEROUS AS SMOKING?

Haven't we always been meat eaters? Well, the answer is yes, if you ask followers of the paleo and Stone Age diets, but no, if you look at research. According to the Stone Age diet, people ate locally available food, and we can be pretty certain that the consumption of meat was limited. The fact that humans can't produce vitamin C, that our teeth are flat, and that our intestines are a bit too long for optimal digestion of meat speaks volumes against the fact that we used to survive primarily on meat. According to the World Health Organization, the WHO, eating less meat is the right thing to do. The WHO claims we should not eat huge amounts of red meat as it can probably cause cancer. We know that processed meats can cause cancer, and the WHO has recently classified consumption of processed meats in the same risk category as smoking, even if smoking is a lot more dangerous. The WHO recommends that we limit the intake of red meat (beef, pork, lamb, and venison) to 1.1 pounds of cooked weight per week. Preferably, processed meats such as sausages, bacon, blood pudding, and pâté should not be eaten at all. This might be news for some of you! Currently three out of four men and almost every second woman in Sweden eat more than this on a regular basis.

My tip: Reduce your consumption of red and processed meats!

RESISTANCE TO ANTIBIOTICS

Antibiotics are not in the meat that we eat. However, it is used in meat production, primarily in animal fodder, to increase growth, which in turn can lead to a resistance to antibiotics and multidrug-resistant bacteria. We definitely don't want this and Sweden was the first country in the world to forbid antibiotics in animal fodder.

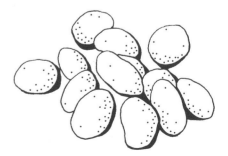

GOOD SOURCES OF PROTEIN FOR THOSE WHO WANT TO EAT VEGETARIAN

The elimination phase

Quinoa

Edamame

Tofu

Rice, all types, preferably wholegrain or brown rice

Buckwheat, teff, and oats

Canned lentils

Quorn

Dairy products

Eggs

Reintroduction phase

Mung beans

Black beans

Canned chickpeas

FIVE VEGETARIAN MYTHS

1. We humans need protein!

Yes, we do. But it doesn't have to be animal protein. Protein from plants is just as good. The most important thing is that you vary and combine sources of vegetable proteins, such as lentils and rice, corn and green leaves, or millet and buckwheat. This means you get all the important amino acids.

2. You can't build muscle without meat.

It's time to debunk the myth that you can't build muscle without meat. Of course you can! It even works really well. The body needs protein—that is, amino acids—but recent studies show that it works just as well if you get protein from vegetarian foods. So you don't need to eat beef to get beefed! Spirulina is a nutrient-rich and FODMAP-friendly protein.

3. Vegetarian food is just strange lentil and bean stews!

Well, these days we have come along a bit when it comes to new, exciting foods and dishes. Vegetarian meals can contain kimchi, bok choy, miso, yuzu, and *furikake*. Sounds both delicious and exciting, doesn't it?

4. You'll be hungry just eating salads!

Of course, salad isn't the best choice when you want to fill up. Fibrous vegetables are filling, however. The crunchier the better. Choose vegetables and root vegetables with care and make sure you vary them. Stomach-friendly legumes such as lentils and chickpeas are very filling, too.

5. It's too expensive to eat fruits and vegetables!

Of course, buying strawberries and melon in the winter is expensive. The key to eating cheap green food is to work with the seasons. Cabbage, carrots, and potatoes are nearly always cheap. Also, buy frozen vegetables and berries, as they contain as many nutrients as fresh ones, sometimes even more.

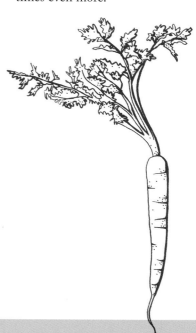

27

Are you getting enough nutrients?

Nutrients are important, and these days it is more important than ever as we are under a lot of stress. Despite this many of us don't get enough nutrients. What is the reason for this? A number of things, including junk food, processed food, unfertile soil, and an increased loss of nutrients caused by stress and exercise. It's impossible for a plant-based product to contain more nutrients than the soil does. Farming on a large scale with a monoculture leads to erosion, and, subsequently, the soil's organic matter reduces, as does the number of earthworms and microorganisms, which are sensitive to pesticides. Additionally, the bee population is declining, and bees struggle to find food. So could it be that we eat more because the body lacks important nutrients?

My tip: Choose locally produced foods, grow your own, choose organic if you can, and if you want to be a real hero, get a beehive.

IRON

Iron is an important mineral that is needed for blood production and therefore transportation of oxygen in the body. Too little iron and we get tired and lack energy. Those with a sensitive stomach know that iron supplements can make your stomach even worse.

My tip: Try and get iron through diet instead.

FODMAP:

- *Pumpkin seeds*
- *Mung beans*
- *Lentils*
- *Spelt flour*
- *Sesame seeds*
- *Oat and bran*
- *Blueberries*
- *Tofu*
- *Sunflower seeds*
- *Dark chocolate (!)*

MAGNESIUM

It doesn't matter if you eat vegetarian food or not, we all need magnesium, no question. We lose magnesium when we are stressed or overexercised, and it is hard to get large amounts through diet alone, especially if you are following a FODMAP diet. Magnesium is good for constipation, if you struggle with sleep, and if you suffer from osteoporosis.

My tip: Magnesium citrate and magnesium oxide are especially good for constipation. Take a supplement in the evening.

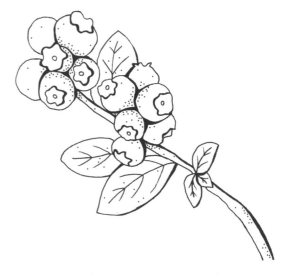

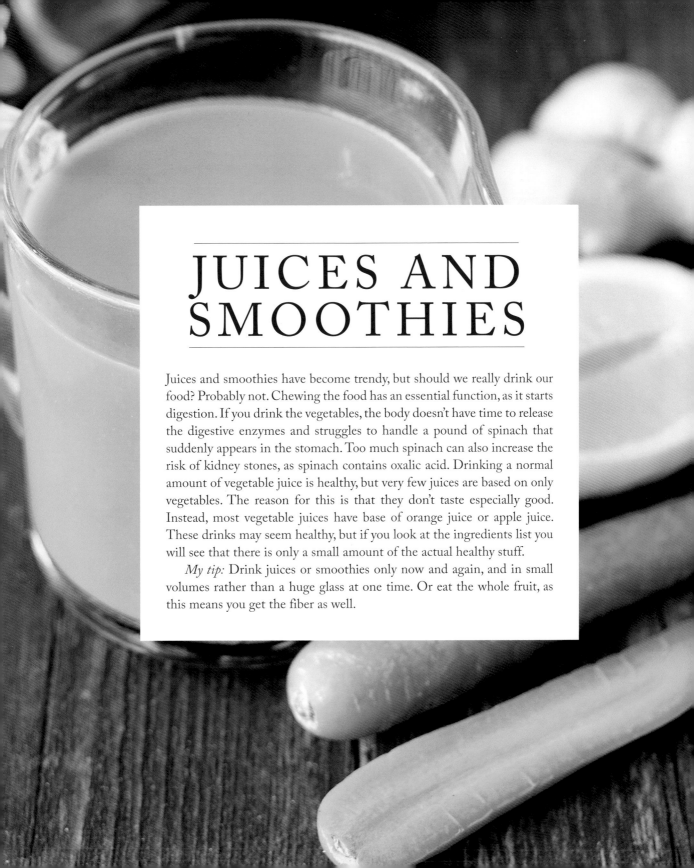

JUICES AND SMOOTHIES

Juices and smoothies have become trendy, but should we really drink our food? Probably not. Chewing the food has an essential function, as it starts digestion. If you drink the vegetables, the body doesn't have time to release the digestive enzymes and struggles to handle a pound of spinach that suddenly appears in the stomach. Too much spinach can also increase the risk of kidney stones, as spinach contains oxalic acid. Drinking a normal amount of vegetable juice is healthy, but very few juices are based on only vegetables. The reason for this is that they don't taste especially good. Instead, most vegetable juices have base of orange juice or apple juice. These drinks may seem healthy, but if you look at the ingredients list you will see that there is only a small amount of the actual healthy stuff.

My tip: Drink juices or smoothies only now and again, and in small volumes rather than a huge glass at one time. Or eat the whole fruit, as this means you get the fiber as well.

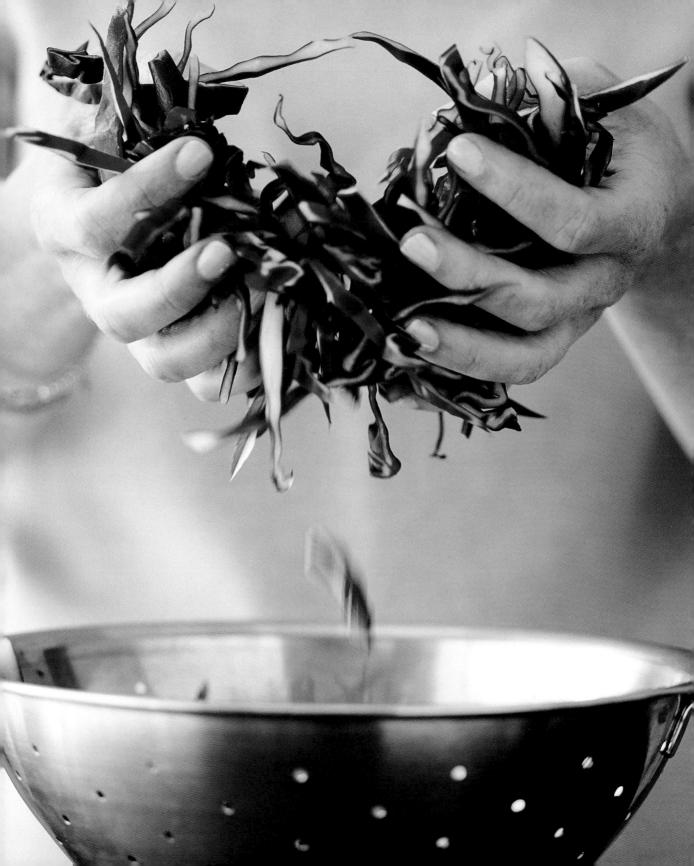

31

CAN WE TALK FOOD WASTE?

If everyone lived the way the Swedes do, we would need 4.2 planets. It's therefore high time we eat our food and save resources. Swedes throw away an average of 163 pounds of food per person a year, and around sixty-two pounds of this is fit to eat. That says something about the "throwaway" mentality when it comes to food.

We are probably influenced by the "best-before" dates, instead of smelling and tasting the food, plus we don't plan our meals as much as we did in previous generations. What we are maybe having for dinner can wait while we get takeout. Fruit and vegetables get thrown away in the largest amounts, so it is really time to consider what we are doing and eat what we buy.

Here are some tips:
- *Juice vegetables and fruits that are starting to turn.* Often, they have flavor just when they are starting to turn, and don't taste as good eaten as they are. Grated vegetables can be used in cooking and baking.

- *Plan!* It sounds boring, but if you embrace the meal planning mentality and make sure what you buy can be used for several meals over the week, you reduce waste. Smell, taste, and look at food rather than checking the "best-before" date and throwing it away. Many times food keeps a lot longer than the date on the packaging. There are, of course, things that should never be eaten after their "sell by" date, but they are usually animal products.

About the recipes

All recipes are adapted to a FODMAP diet, which means they don't use onion, garlic, some seeds, and lactose. Sometimes it uses limited foods. You need to avoid them if you are in the elimination phase, and after that you can decide if you can eat them and how much or if you want to swap it for a different food.

- *Scallions/Leeks.* They are the stomach's best friend. As the fiber—oligosaccharides—is found in the white part of the onion, you should only use the green part of the scallion or leek. It is not always clear where to stop when chopping these up, so if you are in the elimination phase, just use the dark green part and after that you can move to the light green.

- *Onion and garlic.* The fiber in onion and garlic is released in water, which means that you shouldn't use them in water-based food such as stews, soups, and sauces. You can, however, fry garlic in oil, remove the bits, and then use the oil. You can also buy ready-made garlic oil. On www.bellybalance .se you can buy our concentrated garlic oil. You only need about four drops per portion.

- *Ramson.* The herb lends a great taste of garlic to food.

- *Vegetarian alternatives.* In this book you won't find many of these, but of course you can add these if you wish. Tofu, tempeh, seitan, and Quorn are all FODMAP friendly. There's more about soy on the next page.

- *Cereals.* Oats and spelt are two cereals that are used in this book. Both are allowed during the elimination phase. Wheat, rye, and corn are not allowed during the elimination phase.

- *Legumes.* Use ready-cooked legumes in Tetra Paks or cans. The fiber in legumes—oligosaccharides—is water soluble and dissolves in the brine. When you remove the liquid and rinse the legumes, they are better for your gut. Lentils, chickpeas, black beans, and mung beans are all good alternatives. Most other beans have too many oligosaccharides to start with.

- *Soy.* Soy is different as it is classed both as high and low FODMAP. The green soybean edamame is fine, but yellow soybeans are high FODMAP. Soy sauce is fermented and therefore okay to eat, as is tofu because it is pressed, which removes the fiber in the process.

To make it easier for vegans, I have marked the recipes that are vegan. Otherwise I will give suggestions on how to make the recipe vegan if possible.

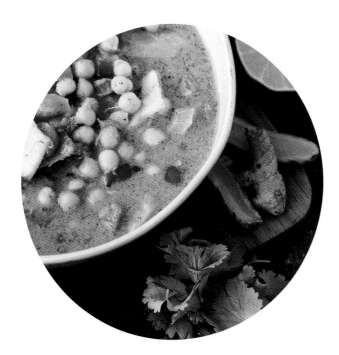

VEGETABLE STOCK

We use an onion-free stock in the recipes. You can make your own vegetable stock with this recipe.

2 carrots
4 potatoes
½ celeriac
1 leek (the green part)
1 parsnip
Around 2 pints of water
3 bay leaves
10 black peppercorns
2 teaspoons salt
Dried herbs (e.g. oregano, thyme, and rosemary)

INSTRUCTIONS

1. Peel and finely chop the carrots, potatoes, celeriac, and parsnips. Place in a large casserole and add enough water to cover the vegetables, around 2 pints.
2. Add bay leaves, peppercorns, salt, and herbs and leave to simmer under a lid on low heat for around 2 hours. Use a spoon to press the vegetables against the bottom of the pan to get more flavor out. Pour the mixture through a sieve and retain the stock.
3. Leave to boil without a lid until the liquid is reduced by half and the stock becomes concentrated. Leave to cool and then pour into ice cube trays and store in the freezer.

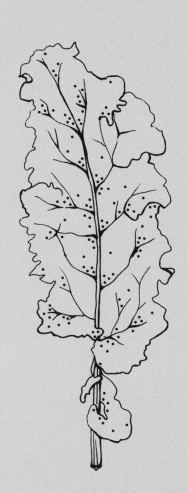

Smoothies, bowls, & bars

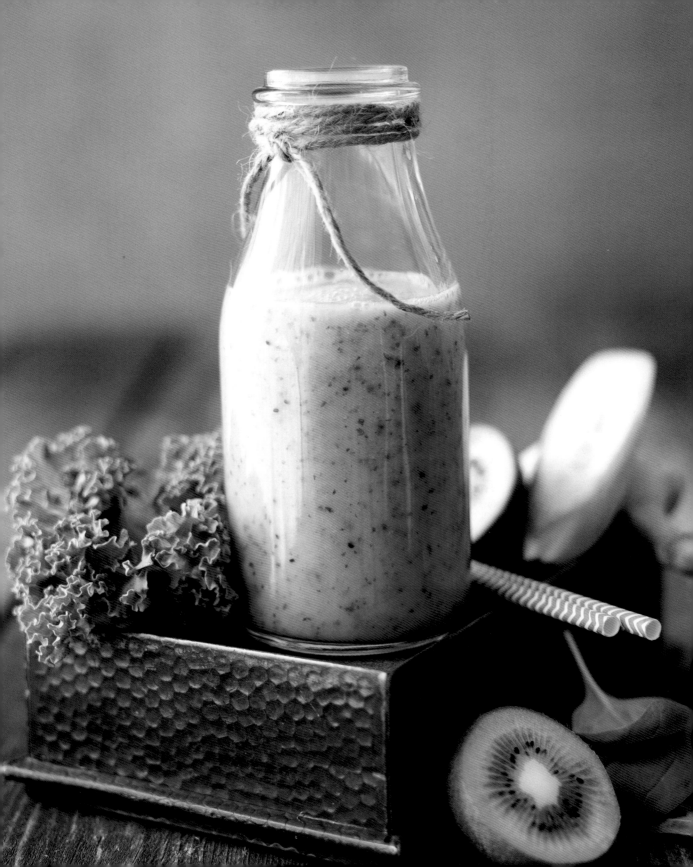

This smoothie contains lots of prebiotic fiber, which nourishes our gut bacteria, and we need to look after those. Feed them the right food and in return they will keep you healthy and happy. Vegan? Choose oat yogurt instead.

BELLY BALANCE SMOOTHIE

SERVES 1

2 kiwifruit
1 lime
½ banana
1 handful of spinach
2 tablespoons oats
⅔ cup lactose-free yogurt
⅓ cup freshly squeezed orange
   juice

INSTRUCTIONS

1. Peel the kiwifruit, lime, and banana.
2. Mix everything together and blend to make a smoothie.

TIPS

If you are in the elimination phase, just drink half a glass.

Ginger is essentially the root of all good. It's been called anti-inflammatory, as it has the ability to reduce inflammation in the body. In addition, it is great for digestion. Drink a shot every day!

38
*Smoothies,
bowls & bars*

GINGER KICK

MAKES ABOUT 1¼ CUPS

1 lemon
1–2 inches fresh ginger
7 carrots

INSTRUCTIONS

1. Remove the peel from the lemon, making sure you remove the white pith that can otherwise give a sour taste.
2. Peel the ginger and carrots if you like. Place in a blender (cut into smaller pieces first) or press through a juice machine.
3. Pour into glasses and serve immediately.

TIPS

Slice the ginger, place in a cup, and pour boiling water on top. Perfect for an evening tea.

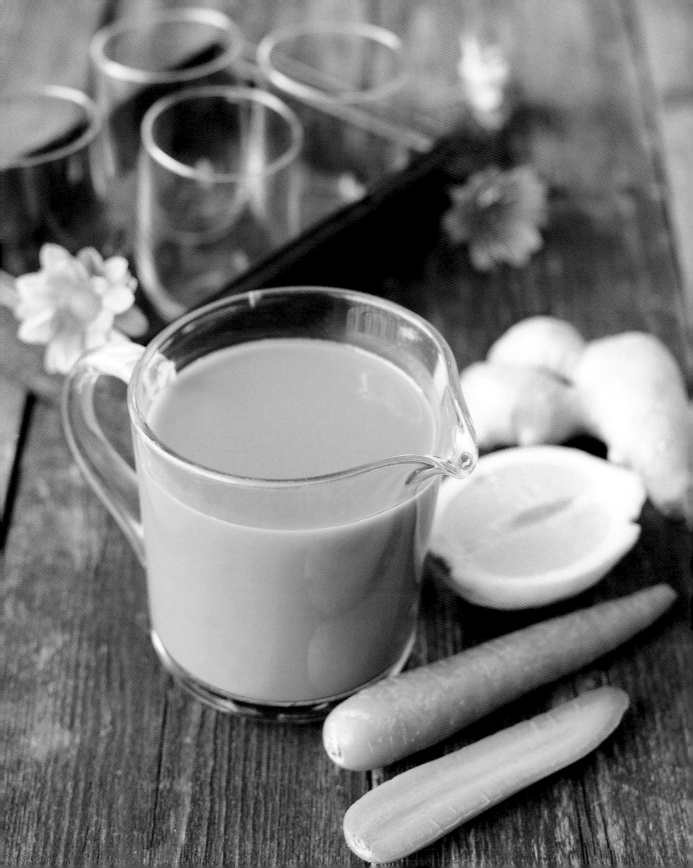

Spirulina is a super algae rich in phycocyanins, which protect the body's cells. It also contains chlorophyll, protein, vitamins, and minerals that are extra important if you have a vegetarian or vegan diet. If you have reintroduced avocado, it makes a nice addition to this smoothie.

BLUEBERRY AND SPIRULINA SMOOTHIE

SERVES 1

1 banana
⅕ cup frozen raspberries
⅖ cup frozen blueberries
¼ avocado (for those who can eat it)
1 lemon, pressed juice
2 teaspoons spirulina powder
⅘ cup almond milk

INSTRUCTIONS

1. Mix all the ingredients in a food processor or use a stick blender.
2. Pour into a glass and enjoy.

TIPS

Store-bought almond milk only contains 2 percent almond and is therefore okay to use.

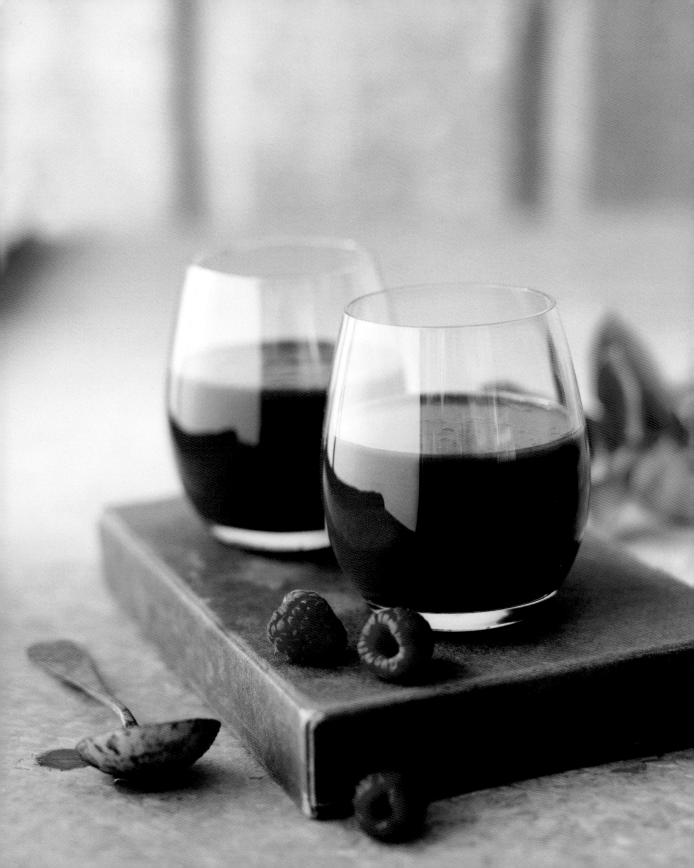

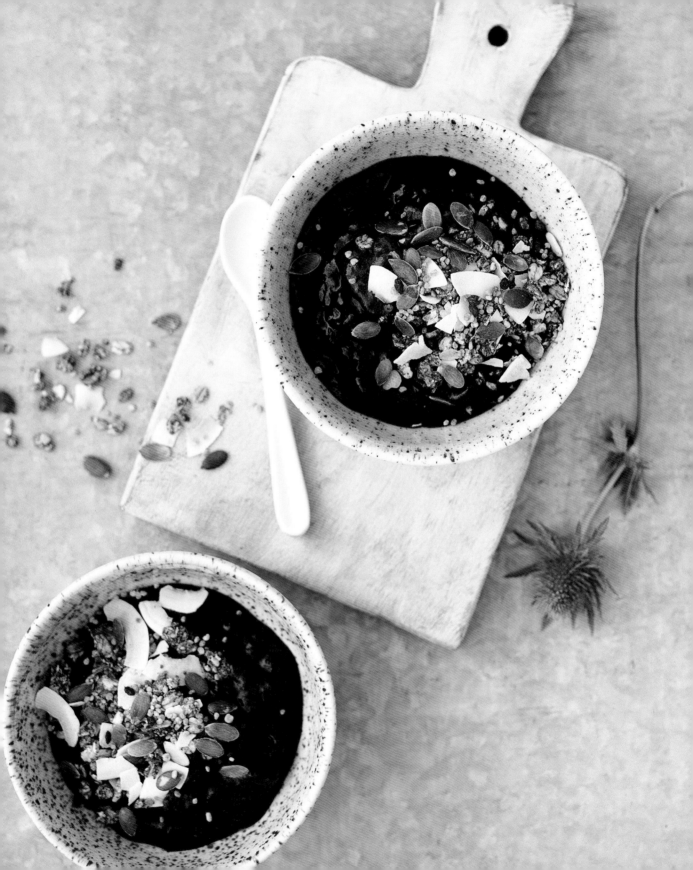

*Blueberries are really healthy and also gentle on the gut.
Here they are mixed with acai, which is also rich in
nutrients. If you can't find acai, just blueberries are fine.*

BLUEBERRY BOWL

SERVES 1

Bowl
⅘ cup frozen blueberries
1 banana
1 tablespoon acai powder (optional)

Topping
Fresh blueberries
Fresh raspberries
Roasted coconut chips
Passion fruit
Gut-friendly granola

INSTRUCTIONS

1. Mix the blueberries, banana, and
   acai powder with a stick blender.
2. Pour into a bowl and top off with
   your blueberries, raspberries,
   coconut chips, and passion fruit. If
   you have some gut-friendly granola
   at home, you can also add this.
3. Serve immediately.

TIPS

*At bellybalance.se,
you can find recipes for
gut-friendly granola.*

A lovely bowl full of healthy things such as spinach and green cabbage as well as avocado if you can eat it. If you can't eat peanuts, you can use walnut butter instead.

44

*Smoothies,
bowls & bars*

SUPERGREEN SMOOTHIE BOWL

SERVES 1

Bowl
¼ avocado (if you can eat it)
1 banana, frozen and sliced
⅓ cup frozen strawberries
⅓ cup frozen raspberries
1 large handful of spinach
½ handful of kale with stalks
    removed
½ tablespoon flaxseeds
1 tablespoon salted peanut butter
⅘ cup almond milk

Topping
Roasted sunflower seeds or
    pumpkin seeds
Gut-friendly granola
Roasted nuts (almond, pecans,
    walnuts)
Coconut chips
Fresh berries
Kiwifruit
Banana
Baby spinach

INSTRUCTIONS

1. Mix all the ingredients to a
   smooth and creamy consistency.
2. Add more almond milk if you
   need it.
3. Pour into a bowl and top
   off with some or all of the
   suggestions to the left.

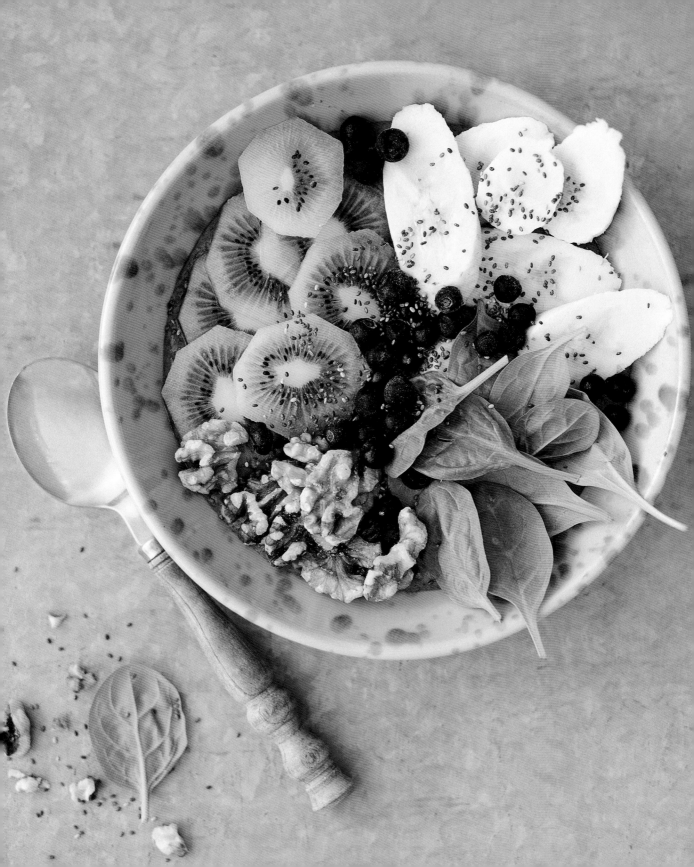

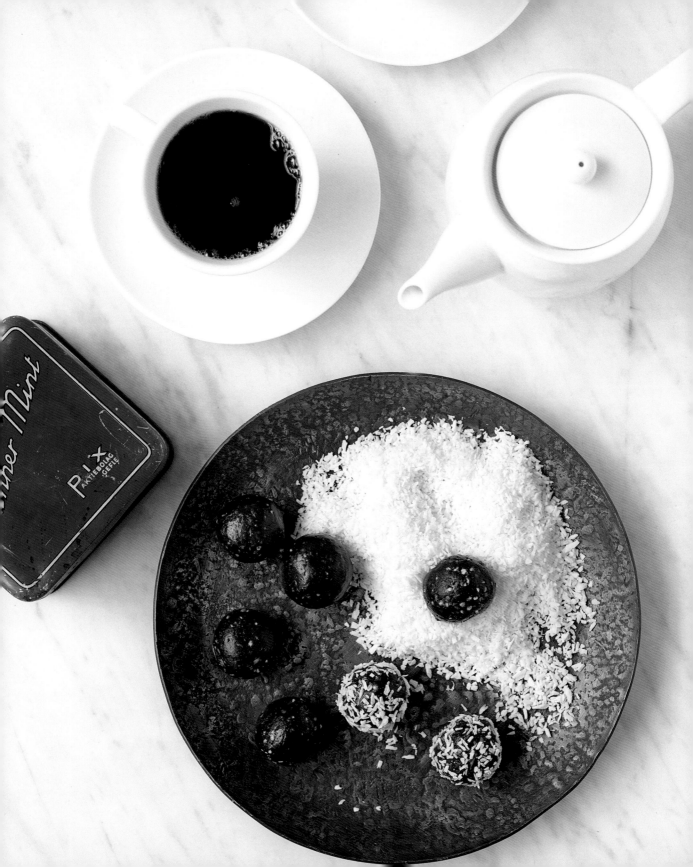

Tasty balls are perfect as a snack, or as a healthy alternative with your coffee. Take some with you when you visit people, and you will always have something that is gentle on your gut to eat.

ENERGY BALLS

MAKES AROUND 15

½ cup nut butter (such as peanut or walnut)
⅕ cup cocoa powder
⅕ cup light syrup
⅖ quinoa puffs
⅓ cup chopped hazelnuts or walnuts
Desiccated coconut (optional)

INSTRUCTIONS

1. Mix the nut butter, cocoa, and syrup. Add the quinoa puffs and chopped nuts.
2. Mix together with a spoon and then use your hands to shape into balls that can be rolled in the coconut. Place in the fridge and remove them just before serving.

TIPS

If you can't find quinoa puffs, you can use rice puffs or oats.

Pop in your bag and eat when you feel your energy levels are dipping. They are also perfect to eat before or after exercise. Store in the fridge or freezer and make a big batch so you always have some in stock. No funny ingredients, just healthy stuff!

RAW BARS

MAKES 10 TO 12 BARS

⅗ cups pumpkin seeds
⅖ cup dried cranberries
⅖ cup dried strawberries or
　blueberries
2 tablespoons maple syrup
⅘ cup oats
3 tablespoons chia seeds
1–2 tablespoons water
½ teaspoon ground ginger
½ teaspoon ground cinnamon

INSTRUCTIONS

1. Roughly chop pumpkin seeds, dried cranberries, and strawberries/blueberries. Mix with the syrup, oats, chia seeds, water, ginger, and cinnamon, or mix all the ingredients in a food processor.
2. Place some parchment paper in a dish (8x8 inches) and spread the mix to make an even layer. Place a bit of parchment paper on top and gently press the mixture to make it smooth and compact.
3. Place the dish in the fridge for 1 hour. Once cold, cut into pieces. Wrap the pieces in greaseproof paper and store in the fridge or freezer.
4. The bars will keep fresh in the fridge for about two weeks. In the freezer they keep for around two months.

NEED EXTRA PROTEIN?

If you want bars that are slightly denser, mix all the ingredients in a food processor, add two egg whites, smooth into an oven-safe dish, and bake in the oven for 35 to 40 minutes at 500°F. Note that this will make them non-vegan.

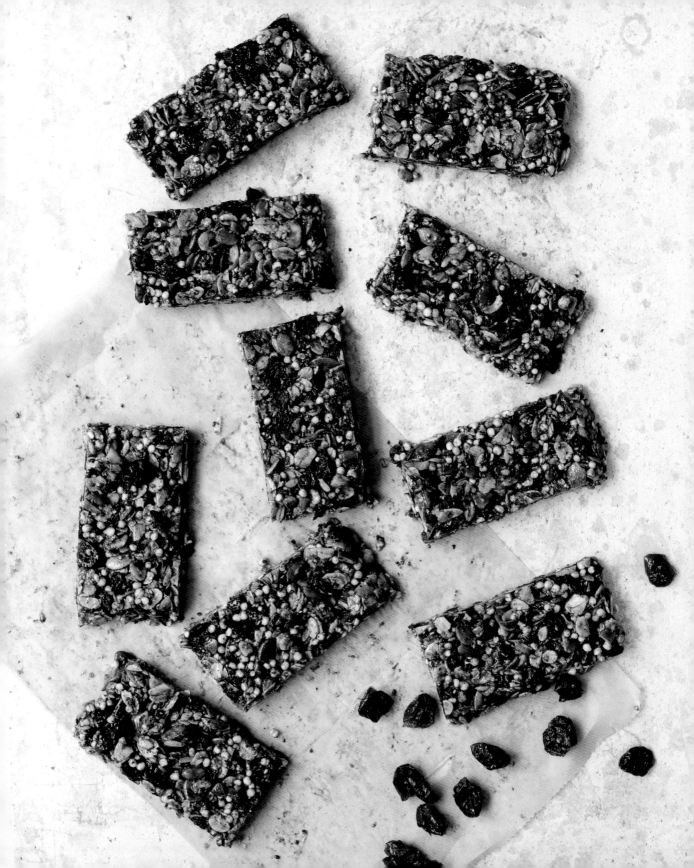

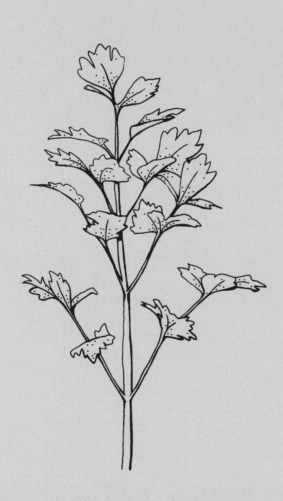

Salads
& soups

This salad contains some ingredients that might be off-limits for some folks. But we are all different, so choose the ingredients that you can handle, depending on how far you've gotten on the diet.

CABBAGE SALAD WITH LINGONBERRY DRESSING

SERVES 4

⅘ cups frozen lingonberries
20 small fresh or frozen brussels
    sprouts
6⅓ pints water
½ pound red cabbage
Olive oil
Flaked salt
1 orange, juice and zest
2 tablespoons maple syrup
1 tablespoon red wine vinegar
⅕ cup olive oil
1 carton chickpeas, ⅗ pound
Salt and black pepper
⅔ cup hazelnuts
½ bunch parsley
Beetroot shoots, optional
Pea shoots, optional

INSTRUCTIONS

1. Thaw the lingonberries and brussels sprouts if you need to. Bring the water to a boil in a saucepan. Finely shred the red cabbage. Remove the outer leaves of the brussels sprouts if they are fresh, and then halve them. Fry for a few minutes in some oil and sprinkle a pinch of flaked salt over it. Place the red cabbage in a colander and pour the hot water over it. Leave for a few minutes. Rinse in cold water and press all the water out.

2. Mix the lingonberries, orange juice, orange zest, maple syrup, vinegar, and olive oil to make a dressing.

3. Rinse the chickpeas thoroughly and mix with the red cabbage and brussels sprouts. Fold the cabbage mix into the dressing and season to taste with salt and pepper. Place on a large serving platter. Roast the hazelnuts in a dry frying pan on medium heat and roughly chop.

4. Chop the parsley. Sprinkle this and the hazelnuts over the cabbage salad. Garnish with beetroot and pea shoots (optional).

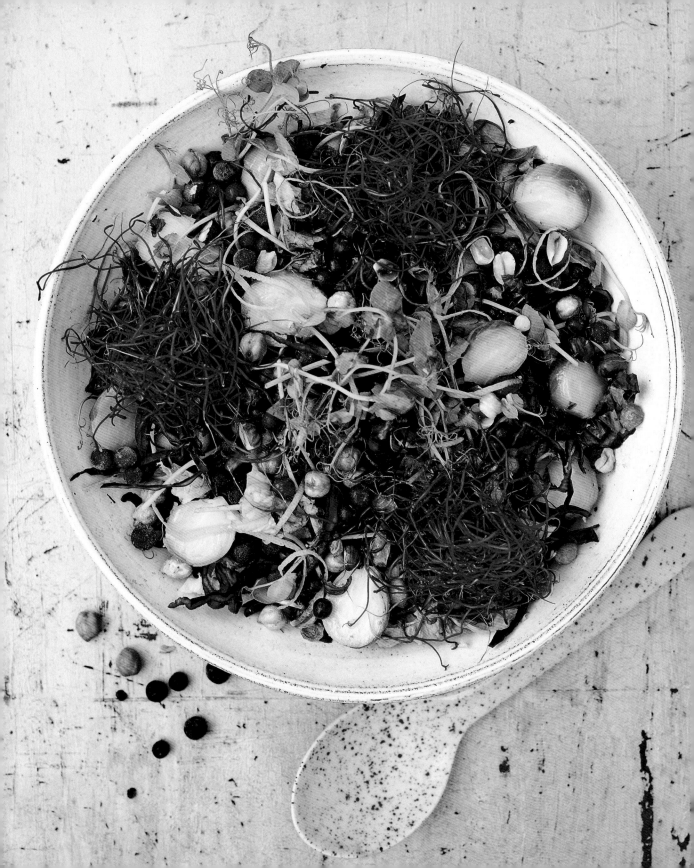

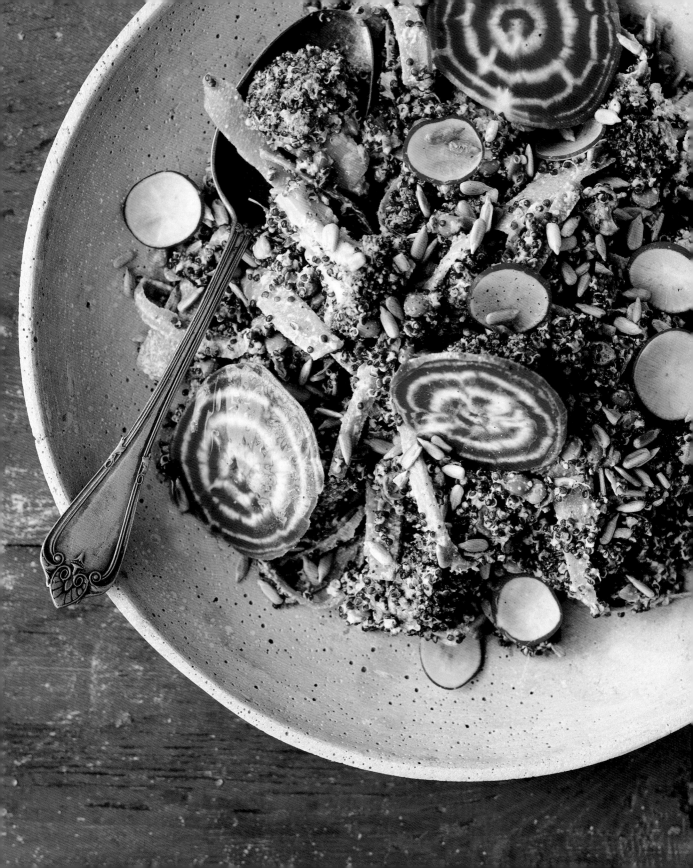

Quinoa is a great staple to have in the FODMAP cupboard. Frozen broccoli is gentler on the stomach than fresh broccoli. Chioggia beet is used mostly as a complement to quinoa because it looks good as a garnish, and you can eat a few slices without any problems.

CREAMY QUINOA SALAD

SERVES 4

Cranberry cream
1¾ ounces dried cranberries
⅔ cup macadamia nuts or roasted sunflower seeds
⅔ cup water
1 tablespoon white balsamic vinegar
1-2 tablespoons olive oil
Salt
Freshly ground pepper

Salad
4 portions of red quinoa
2 carrots
7 ounces frozen broccoli
5 leaves kale
½ bunch parsley
1 bunch radishes
1 Chioggia beet
3 tablespoons sunflower seeds

INSTRUCTIONS

1. Mix cranberries, macadamia nuts or sunflower seeds, and water to make a cream using a mixer or a stick blender. Add white balsamic vinegar, olive oil, salt, and pepper to taste.
2. Cook the quinoa according the instructions on the package. Leave to completely cool.
3. Peel the carrots and shave into ribbons. Thaw the broccoli and cut into small florets. Remove the hard stalks from the kale and shred into smaller pieces. Roughly chop the parsley. Cut the radishes into quarters and thinly slice the Chioggia beet.
4. Roast the sunflower seeds in a dry frying pan. Mix the quinoa with the cranberry cream. Fold in the vegetables and parsley. Garnish with sunflower seeds and the Chioggia beet.

Root vegetables are almost all great for the gut. Sweet potato is okay in smaller amounts, but you can also replace it with normal potato. If you are vegan, replace the goat cheese with a vegan alternative.

56
Salads & soups

WARM SALAD WITH ROOT VEGETABLES AND GOAT CHEESE

SERVES 4

3 carrots

3 parsnips

1 large sweet potato

Some olive oil for the root vegetables

2 tablespoons rosemary, fresh and finely chopped

Salt

3½ ounces savoy cabbage

1 ounce pine nuts

2½ ounces mangold

3½ ounces goat cheese (with a lactose content of max 1g/100 g)

2 tablespoons maple syrup

2 tablespoons olive oil

INSTRUCTIONS

1. Heat the oven to 500°F.
2. Rinse and peel the carrots, parsnips, and sweet potato and cut into small sticks.
3. Mix olive oil and rosemary in a large bowl and fold in the root vegetables. Then place them on a pan with parchment paper and lightly salt. Roast in the oven for around 20 to 30 minutes or until they are soft.
4. Roughly shred the savoy cabbage and quickly fry in a hot pan with some olive oil. Roast the pine nuts in a dry frying pan.
5. Leave the root vegetables to slightly cool. and mix them with the savoy cabbage and mangold. Place the salad on a large serving platter, crumble some goat cheese on top and finish off with roasted pine nuts. Whisk together the maple syrup and 2 tablespoons of olive oil and drizzle over the salad.

TIPS

Save any leftovers for a packed lunch.

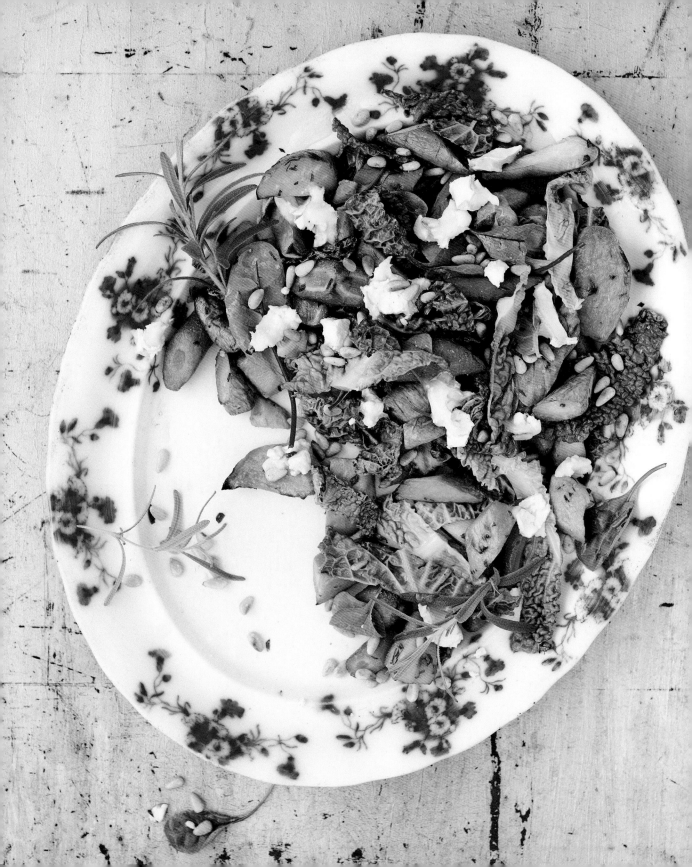

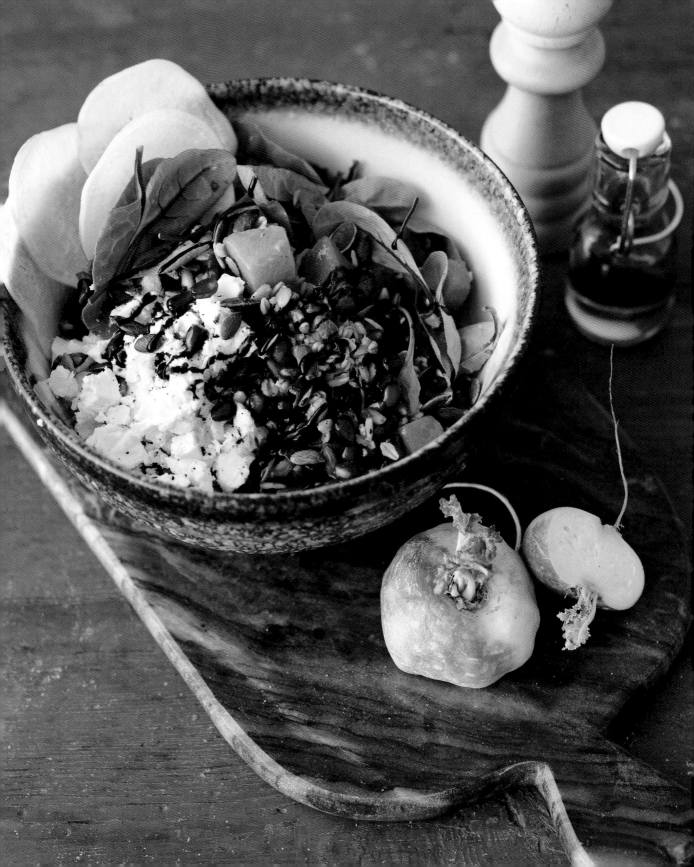

If you can't find Muscat or Hokkaido squash, you can use a smaller amount of butternut squash. Barley is a fiber-rich alternative to rice. Vegan? Replace the feta cheese with a vegan substitute.

ROASTED SQUASH SALAD WITH BARLEY

SERVES 4

1 Muscat or Hokkaido squash
Salt
Freshly ground pepper
Olive oil
2 portions of barley
1 small turnip
½ pomegranate
⅕ cup pumpkin seeds
4⅕ ounces mangold or baby
    spinach
5⅓ ounces feta cheese (with a
    lactose content of max
    1g/100 g)
Flaked salt
Crema di balsamico

INSTRUCTIONS

1. Heat the oven to 450°F. Cut the squash into wedges and remove the skin and seeds. Cut the flesh into large cubes. Place on a pan and add salt, pepper, and drizzle some olive oil over. Roast in the oven for around 20 minutes.
2. Cook the barley according to the instructions on the packaging. Leave to cool. Thinly slice the turnip, preferably with a mandoline, and place the slices in ice-cold water. Remove the seeds from the pomegranate and roast the pumpkin seeds in a dry frying pan.
3. Place the mangold or baby spinach on a serving platter, and add the barley and roasted squash on top.
4. Top off with crumbled feta cheese, pomegranate seeds, freshly ground black pepper, roasted pumpkin seeds, flaked salt, and crema di balsamico.

TIPS

Remove the seeds from a pomegranate by placing the pomegranate in a bowl with water. The seeds will float to the top.

Kimchi originates from Korea, where it is served as an accompaniment to many meals. The original recipe includes garlic, but we will make it without, of course. If you want the kimchi to ferment more, just leave it for longer.

60
Salads
& soups

KIMCHI

SERVES 4

2⅖ pounds cabbage
⅓ cup salt
2 tablespoons chili pepper
    (dried powder)
1½ tablespoons Asian fish sauce
2 tablespoons grated ginger
⅘ cup finely chopped leeks
    (the green part)
2 teaspoons sugar

INSTRUCTIONS

1. Rinse the cabbage and cut into thick strips. Place in a large bowl and add salt and mix. Place a plate over to weigh it down and leave for at least 5 hours in room temperature but preferably overnight.
2. Carefully rinse the cabbage, leave to drain, and squeeze out excess water. Mix the chili pepper, fish sauce, ginger, leeks, and sugar in a large bowl. Add the cabbage and thoroughly mix. Leave the kimchi to rest for an hour or so to allow the flavors to develop.

FERMENTING KIMCHI

1. Place the kimchi mixture in a glass jar with a tight-fitting lid. Fill it all the way up, pressing down on the cabbage. Place the jar on a plate to catch any leakages.
2. Place the jar in room temperature for 3 to 5 days and then in the fridge. After another 5 days, the kimchi is ready.
3. Store in the fridge to allow the flavor to keep developing.

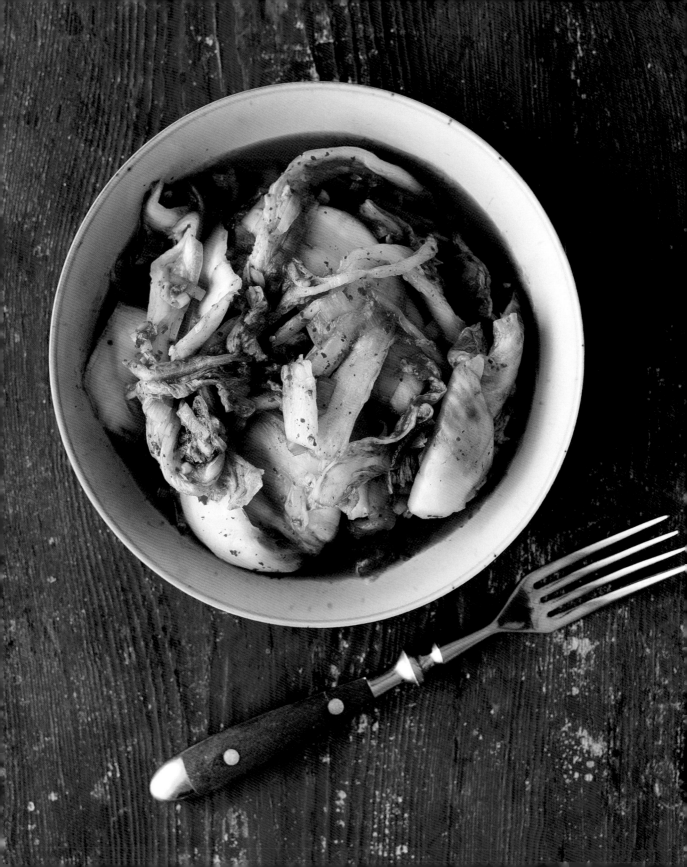

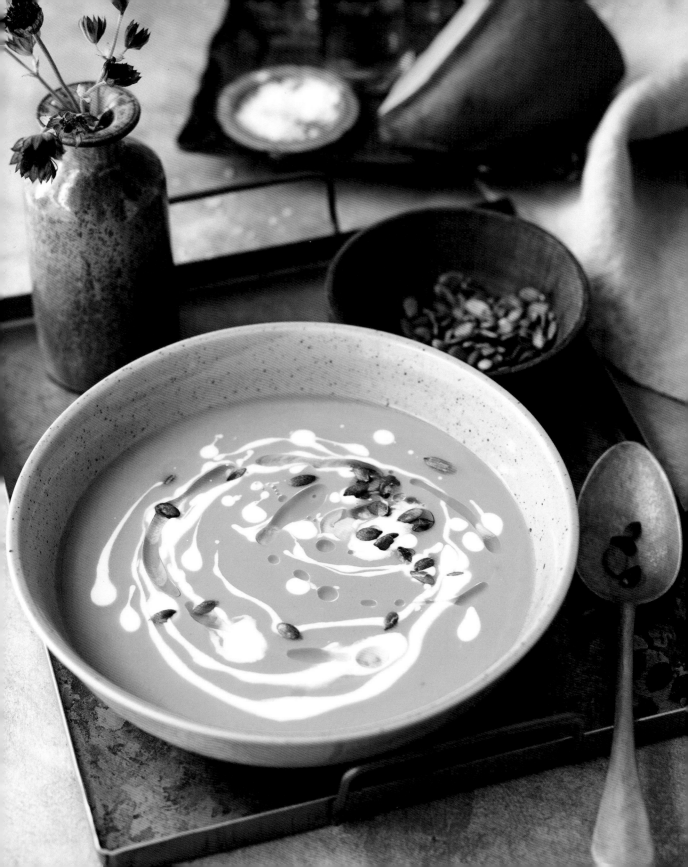

Squash can be found in grocery stores almost year-round. Hokkaido and muscat squash are FODMAP friendly, while butternut squash can be eaten in smaller amounts. You can garnish the soup with crumbled goat cheese. Vegan? Replace the goat cheese with a vegan substitute.

HOT SQUASH SOUP

SERVES 4 TO 6

1½ pound Hokkaido or Muscat
    squash
1⅕ inches ginger
2 scallions (the green part)
1 red chili
1 teaspoon ground cumin
2 tablespoons onion-free
    vegetable stock
2¹⁄₁₀ pints water
1 can coconut milk, ¹⁷⁄₂₀ pint
1 teaspoon concentrated garlic oil
    (optional)
Canola oil
Salt
Freshly ground pepper

To garnish
Pumpkin seeds
Crème fraîche or a vegan alternative
Fresh thyme

INSTRUCTIONS

1. Cut the squash into wedges and
   remove the skin and seeds. Cut
   the flesh into smaller cubes.
2. Peel and finely chop the ginger.
   Finely chop the scallions and
   chili.
3. Fry the squash in canola oil in
   a pot for 4 to 5 minutes. Add
   ginger, scallion, chili, and cumin
   and fry everything for a few
   minutes. Add stock, water, and
   coconut milk. Leave to simmer
   on low heat or until the squash
   is cooked through.
4. Blend the soup with a stick
   blender and season with garlic
   oil, salt, and pepper.
5. Roast the pumpkin seeds in a
   dry frying pan on high heat.
   Drizzle some crème fraîche or
   vegan alternative over the soup.
   Sprinkle pumpkin seeds and
   fresh thyme on top and serve
   with a nice bread.

If you can't get hold of kale, you can also use the same amount of fresh or frozen spinach. Top off the soup with some chopped nuts or seeds, basil, and a drop of cream. Vegan? Skip the eggs and choose rice or oat cream instead.

KALE SOUP

SERVES 4

1⅓ pound kale
2 scallions (the green part)
Butter
2 tablespoons sieves spelt flour
2⅕ pints water
2–3 tablespoons onion-free vegetable stock
⅘ cup lactose-free cream
Salt
White pepper

4 hard-boiled eggs
Freshly ground white pepper

INSTRUCTIONS

1. Rinse the kale and cut off the stalks. Shred the kale and place in a bowl.
2. Finely chop the scallions and fry in some butter in a large saucepan. Add the kale and stir for a minute. Sprinkle over the flour and stir thoroughly. Add water and stock. Stir and leave to cook under a lid for around 20 minutes.
3. Add cream to the soup and season to taste with the salt and white pepper. Serve the soup as it is, or use a stick blender to make it smooth.
4. Serve with egg halves and a piece of bread or cheese, if you like.

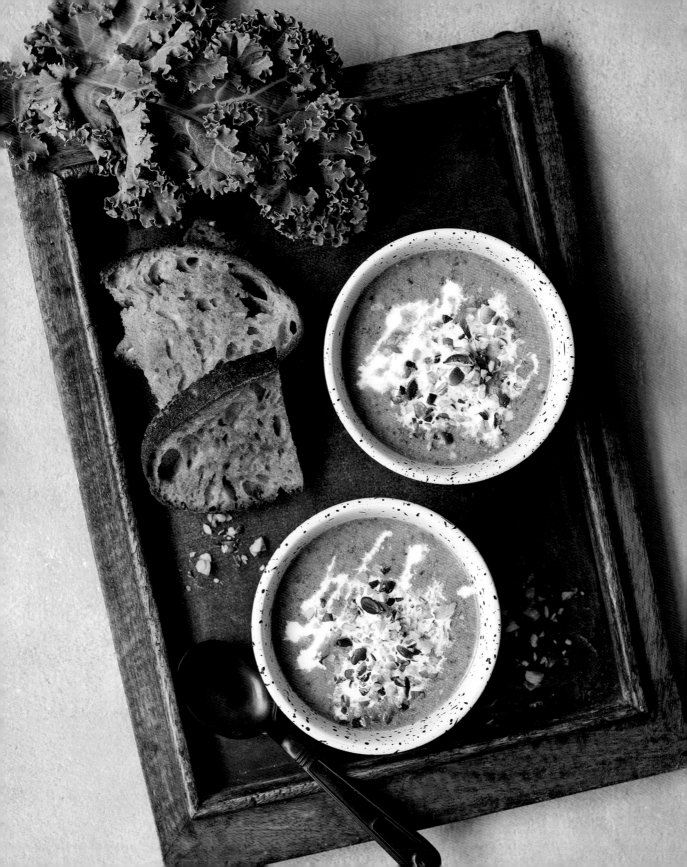

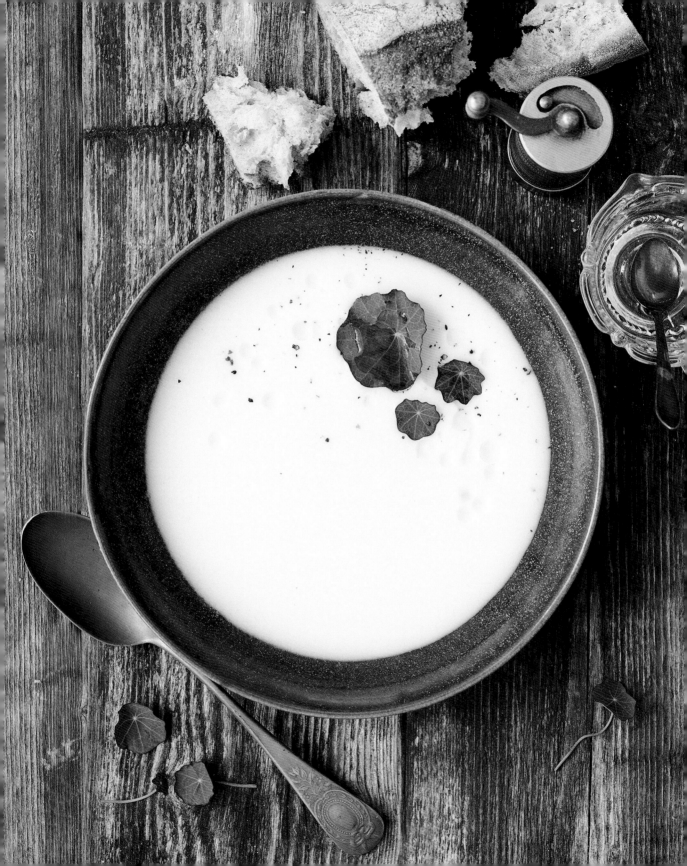

Celeriac is cheap and widely available. The taste is smooth and is perfect for soup. The soup can be frozen so make a large batch while you are at it. Vegan? Replace the cream with rice or oat cream instead.

CREAMY CELERIAC SOUP

SERVES 4

2⅓ pounds celeriac

2 inches ginger

3 carrots

2 scallions (the green part)

1 teaspoon concentrated garlic oil (optional)

Olive oil

2¾ pints water

1¾ cups lactose-free cream

⅓ cup white wine vinegar

2 tablespoons onion-free vegetable stock

1–2 teaspoons soy sauce

1 teaspoon sambal oelek

Salt

INSTRUCTIONS

1. Peel and roughly chop the celeriac, ginger, and carrots. Chop the scallions and fry together with the ginger in garlic oil and olive oil in a large saucepan or casserole dish.

2. Add celeriac and carrots and fry for a few minutes.

3. Add water, cream, white wine vinegar, vegetable stock, soy sauce and sambal oelek. Leave to simmer on low heat under a lid for around 20 minutes.

4. Blend the soup until it is smooth before serving and add salt to taste. Serve with some nice bread.

A smooth soup with a kick depending on how much sambal you use. Black beans are limited to a max of 1¾ ounces (50 grams) and add protein and dietary fiber. Vegan? Use oat fraîche and a vegan alternative to feta cheese.

CARROT AND SAFFRON SOUP

SERVES 4

1¾ pounds carrots
2 scallions (the green part)
2 tablespoons olive oil
1 sachet saffron
½ teaspoon dried thyme
⅘ cup white wine
3⅔ cups water
2 tablespoons onion-free
    vegetable stock
⅘ cup lactose-free crème fraîche
Salt
Black pepper
½ teaspoon sambal oelek
1¾ ounce feta cheese (where the
    lactose content is max 1g/100 g)

Tomato salad
2 tomatoes
7 ounces canned black beans
2 tablespoons olive oil
1 tablespoon balsamic vinegar
Salt
Freshly ground black pepper

INSTRUCTIONS

1. Peel and cut the carrots into smaller pieces. Finely chop the scallions. Heat the oil in a large saucepan and fry the carrots, scallions, saffron, and thyme for around 1 minute. Add the wine and reduce for around 1 minute. Add the water and stock, and leave the soup to simmer under a lid for around 15 minutes or until the carrots are soft.

2. Thinly slice the tomatoes for the salad. Drain the beans and rinse under cold water. Place the tomatoes on a plate and pour over the beans. Drizzle over some oil and vinegar and add salt and pepper.

3. Blend the soup with a stick blender. Add crème fraîche and sambal oelek, salt, and pepper to taste. Crumble feta cheese on top of the soup and serve with the tomato salad.

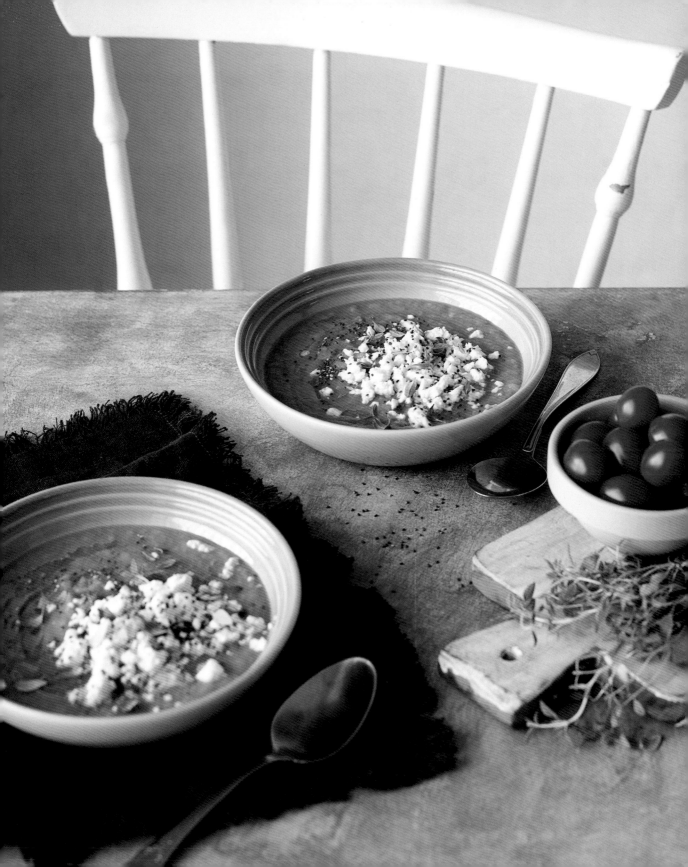

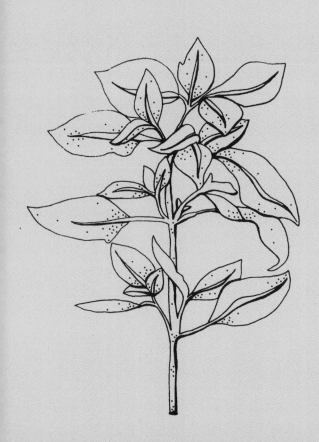

Pasta, risotto & stews

This is a classic Italian dish. Melanzane, *or aubergine gratin, tastes almost better the day after. So make sure you prepare in good time, preferably the day before, and then heat it at 300°F for around 15 minutes. Vegan? Replace the cheese with a vegan alternative.*

MELANZANE ALLA PARMIGIANA

SERVES 4 TO 6

2 aubergines
3–4 tablespoons salt
2 tablespoons olive oil
2 mozzarellas, 4⅖ ounces each (125 gram) (with a lactose content of max 1g/100 g)

Tomato sauce
3 scallions (the green part)
Olive oil
2 cans of cherry tomatoes, 9/10 pound each (400 grams)
1 teaspoon sugar
7 sprigs of oregano (or 1 tablespoon dried)
6 sprigs of thyme (or ½ tablespoon dried)
½ bunch basil
Salt
Freshly ground black pepper

Bread mix
⅘ cup grated vegetarian Parmesan
⅔ cup gluten-free grated white bread
Sourdough bread made from spelt or gluten-free bread crumbs
½ teaspoon salt
1 tablespoon finely chopped parsley
3 tablespoons olive oil

INSTRUCTIONS

1. Heat the oven to 350°F. Slice the eggplant as thinly as you can. Salt the slices and leave them in a colander. Place a weight on top and leave to drain for at least one hour.
2. Make the tomato sauce: chop the scallions and fry in olive oil in a saucepan. Add tomatoes, sugar, herbs, salt, and pepper, and leave to simmer for 10 to 15 minutes.
3. Brush the salt off the aubergines and place the slices close together on a baking pan with parchment paper. Drizzle some olive oil over and bake in the middle of the oven for around ten minutes. Once done, leave them to rest on the parchment paper.
4. Make the bread mix: Grate the vegetarian Parmesan cheese and mix with the bread/bread crumbs, salt, and finely chopped parsley.
5. Thinly slice the mozzarella. Increase the oven temperature to 450°F.
6. Place some of the bread mixture in the bottom of a heat-proof dish. Pour some tomato sauce on top and add a third of the aubergine and mozzarella mix. Keep layering all the ingredients in the same way until you use the whole mix. Top off with some extra Parmesan and olive oil. Place in the middle of the oven for 15 to 20 minutes. Leave to cool slightly before serving. Serve with a salad and some bread.

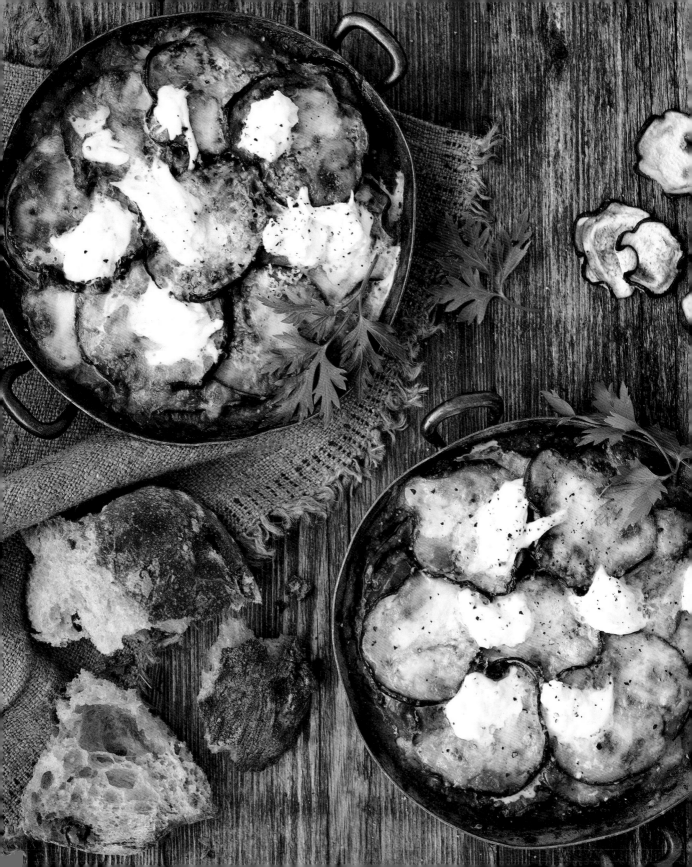

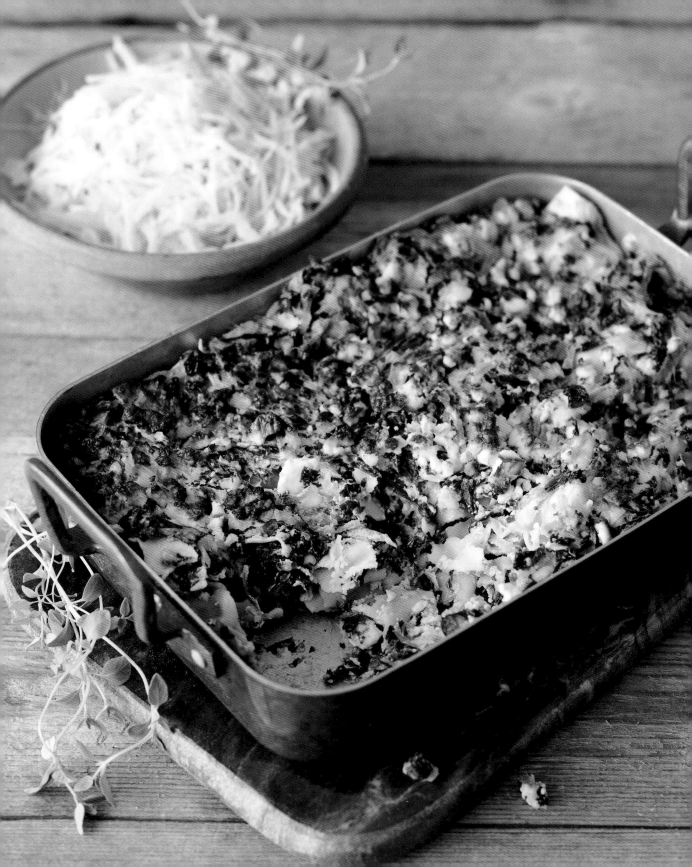

A classic dish with a green twist that can easily be frozen. Gluten-free lasagna can be found in regular grocery stores. Just make sure you choose the ones that don't contain soy flour. Vegan? Replace the cheese with a vegan alternative and use rice or oat milk.

VEGETARIAN LASAGNA

SERVES 4

1 pound frozen chopped spinach
1 large garlic clove
Olive oil
2 scallions (the green part)
2 large carrots
½ pound ricotta cheese
½ pound cottage cheese
3½ ounces feta cheese (where the lactose content is max 1g/100 g)
⅘ cup lactose-free milk
3 pinches grated nutmeg
Salt
Freshly ground black pepper
12 gluten-free lasagna sheets
½ cup strong, grated cheese

Coleslaw
1 pound white cabbage
3 tablespoons canola oil
1 tablespoon white wine vinegar
Salt
Black pepper or French herbs
⅓ cup pickled peppers (optional)

INSTRUCTIONS

1. Heat the oven to 400°F. Thaw the spinach. Peel and cut the garlic clove into pieces (not too small). Heat some olive oil in a large saucepan and fry the garlic until brown. Remove all the garlic bits (don't leave any). Slice the scallions and fry in the same pan for a few minutes. Add the spinach and fry for another few minutes. Remove the saucepan from the heat and leave to cool.

2. Roughly grate the carrots. Mix the spinach with carrots, ricotta, cottage cheese, crumbled feta cheese, milk, nutmeg, salt, and pepper.

3. Place a sheet of lasagna at the bottom of an heatproof dish. Layer the filling with the lasagna and sprinkle grated cheese on top. Bake in the oven for around 30 minutes.

4. Shred the cabbage with a cheese slicer or mandoline. Mix with oil, vinegar, salt, pepper or French herbs, and chopped peppers (optional).

5. Serve the lasagna with the coleslaw.

Meh, where are the vegetables? Okay, so this might not be the healthiest of dishes, but it's definitely one of the tastiest! Butter and pasta will make your reward system jump for joy! You are definitely worth it, so eat this in good faith now and again. Vegan? Use lactose-free butter and a vegan alternative to cheese.

PASTA WITH HOT SAGE BUTTER

SERVES 4

4 servings of gluten-free pasta such
   as linguine
1 red chili
2 scallions (the green part)
3½ ounces butter
20 sage leaves
Flaked salt
Freshly ground black pepper
Vegetarian Parmesan

INSTRUCTIONS

1. Boil the pasta according to
   the instructions on the packet.
   Finely chop the chili and
   scallions. Melt the butter in a
   saucepan until it goes brown
   and has a nutty smell. Remove
   from the heat and add the sage,
   chili, and scallions. Leave for 5
   minutes to infuse.
2. Plate up the pasta and drizzle
   the sage butter on top. Add salt
   and plenty of freshly ground
   pepper and grated vegetarian
   Parmesan. Serve with a nice
   bread.

TIPS

*Butter contains
small amounts of
lactose and does not need
to be lactose free.*

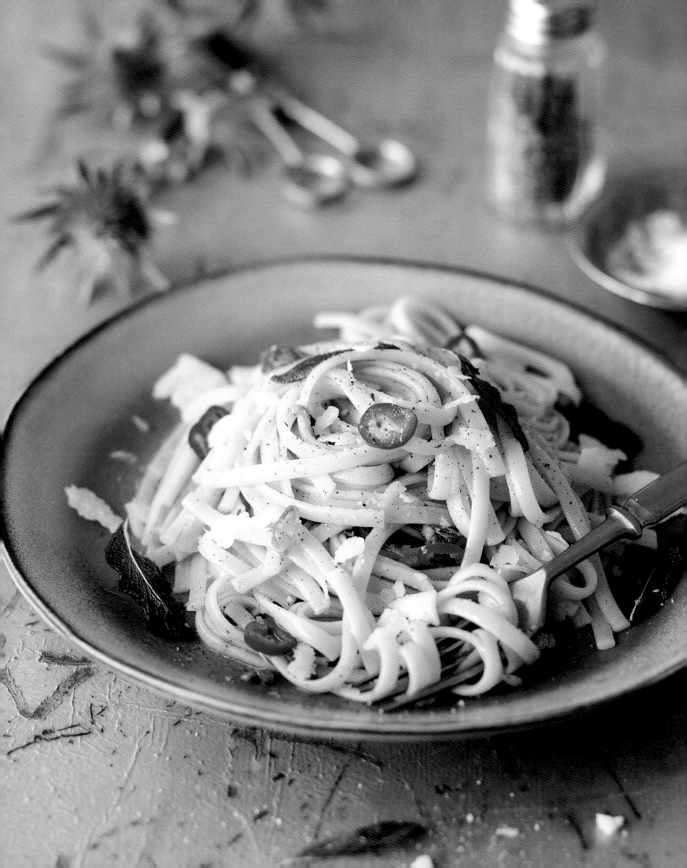

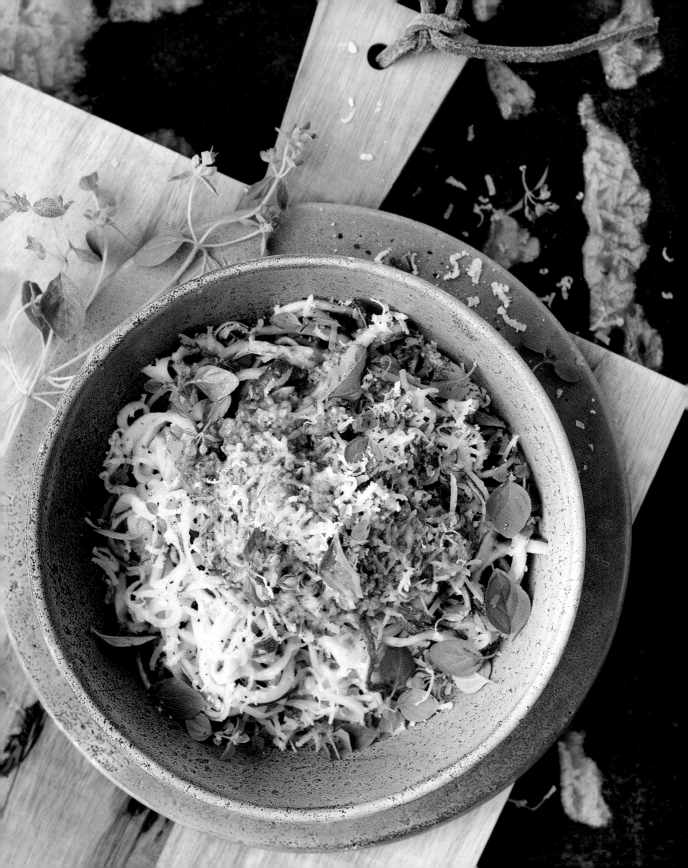

If you want the children to eat more vegetarian food, this is a great dish to start with. Is it Quorn or groundbeef? Kids won't know the difference, promise! Vegan? Use rice or oat cream.

QUORN GROUNDS SAUCE WITH ZUCCHINI PASTA

SERVES 4

3 scallions (the green part)
1 red chili (depending on
    preferred strength)
Butter
½ pound Quorn Grounds
2 tablespoons tomato puree
½ pound crushed tomatoes
1 teaspoon oregano
1 teaspoon rosemary
1 teaspoon basil
1 teaspoon thyme
1 teaspoon ramson
1 tablespoon onion-free vegetable
    stock
⅖ cup of water
⅘ cup lactose-free cream for
    cooking
2 zucchini
Grated cheese
Salt
Freshly ground black pepper

INSTRUCTIONS

1. Finely chop the scallion and
   chili. Melt some butter in a
   frying pan and quickly fry the
   scallion and chili. Add the
   Quorn Grounds and fry while
   stirring to make it crumbly.
2. Mix in the tomato puree and
   fry for a few minutes. Add
   crushed tomatoes, salt, pepper,
   herbs, and vegetable stock. Stir
   and then leave to simmer for
   around 10 minutes. Add ⅖ cup
   of water if you need to.
3. Add the cream and more herbs
   to taste. Leave to simmer for
   6 to 8 minutes.
4. Boil some water in a saucepan.
   Shred the zucchini lengthwise
   with a cheese slicer or potato
   peeler. Boil the shreds for

1 to 2 minutes and then discard
   the water.
5. Serve the Quorn Grounds
   with the zucchini pasta, grated
   cheese, and a nice salad.

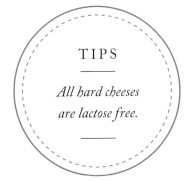

TIPS

*All hard cheeses
are lactose free.*

Making gnocchi sounds a bit pretentious, but it is actually quite easy. One tip is to make double the amount of pesto and save in the fridge. It's great with pasta or on a sandwich. Vegan? Skip the egg and choose a vegan alternative for cheese.

CARROT GNOCCHI WITH CORIANDER PESTO

SERVES 4

Pesto
1 bunch coriander
1 teaspoon concentrated garlic oil
1 tablespoon roasted pine nuts
2 tablespoons olive oil
Freshly ground black pepper

Gnocchi
5 potatoes
3 carrots
1 egg
⅗ cup sieved spelt flour
2 tablespoons finely grated
    Parmesan or pecorino
Black pepper
1 pinch nutmeg (optional)
Grated cheese to serve

INSTRUCTIONS

1. Mix coriander with garlic oil, roasted pine nuts, and olive oil. Season with black pepper and make a paste. Add more olive oil if you need it. Place the pesto in a jar and place in the fridge.
2. Peel and boil the potatoes and carrots until they are soft. (Cut them into pieces and they boil faster.) Discard the water and leave to cool. Mash the potatoes and carrots with a fork to make a smooth paste. Add egg, flour, grated cheese, black pepper, and nutmeg. Mix with your hands to make a smooth dough. If the dough is sticky, you can add more flour.
3. Divide the dough into four balls. On a floured surface, roll each ball to make a long sausage and cut into ¾-inch-thick pieces. Gently press each gnocchi with a fork to make a pattern.
4. Boil some lightly salted water in a large saucepan. Carefully place 10 gnocchi in the pan and boil for 30 seconds—the gnocchi will float to the top when they are done. Remove with a skimmer spoon and place in a pre-warmed dish. Mix in a teaspoon of pesto. Add a new batch of gnocchi to the saucepan and repeat until all the gnocchi is done.
5. Serve with grated cheese and a green salad.

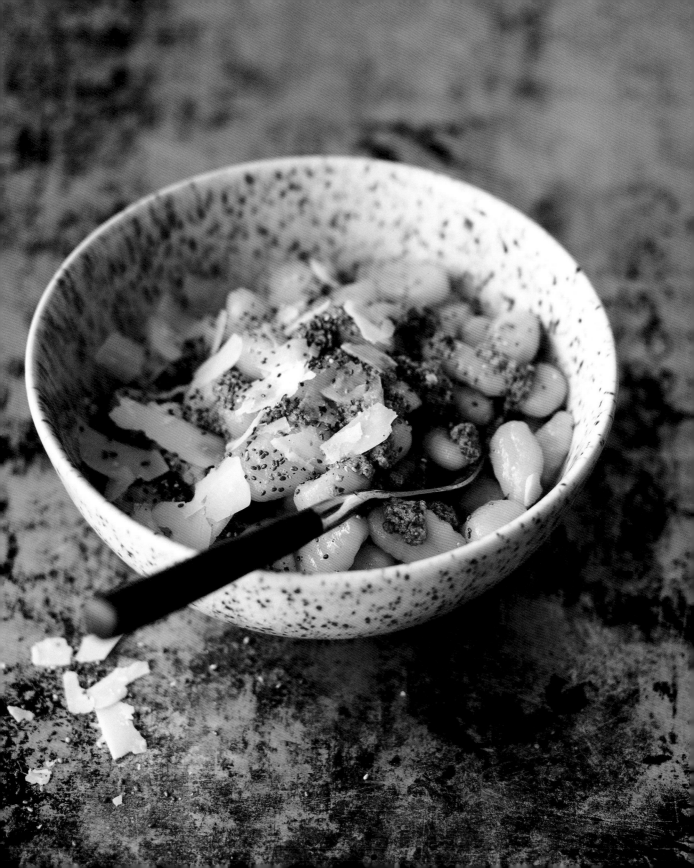

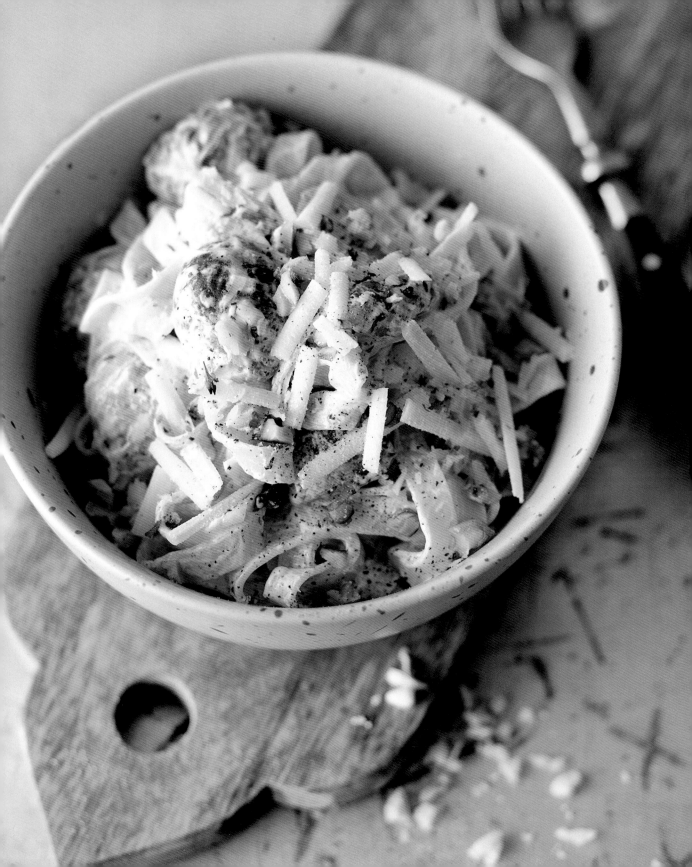

*You can use either cream or crème fraîche here—both
work. If you are sensitive to fat, you can choose products
with a lower fat content. You can also use kale instead
of brussels sprouts. Vegan? Use oat or rice cream and a
vegan alternative to cheese.*

CREAMY BRUSSELS SPROUTS PASTA

SERVES 4

Just under 1 pound pasta, such as
tagliatelle (400 gram)
2 scallions (the green part)
½ pound brussels sprouts
1 teaspoon dried ramson
2 tablespoons olive oil
1½ cups lactose-free cream or
crème fraîche
4 tablespoons pine nuts
1¾ ounce grated vegetarian
Parmesan (around ⅖ cup)
1 teaspoon lemon zest plus some
to garnish
1 tablespoon lemon juice
Flaked salt
Freshly ground black pepper

INSTRUCTIONS

1. Boil the pasta according to the
instructions on the package.
Finely chop the scallions.
Defrost the brussels sprouts and
halve them. Fry the scallion and
ramson in olive oil for a few
minutes in a frying pan. Add
the brussels sprouts and fry for
another 3 minutes. Add cream
or crème fraîche and cook until
blended.
2. Roast the pine nuts in a dry
frying pan.
3. Discard the water from the
pasta. Mix the pasta with
the brussels sprouts mixture,
grated Parmesan, lemon zest,
and lemon juice. Add salt and
pepper to taste.
4. Garnish with pine nuts, lemon
zest, and shaved vegetarian
Parmesan.

TIPS

*Parboil fresh brussels
sprouts to make them
gentler on your gut.*

This is a dish with lots of steps, but well worth the effort as it tastes fantastic. You can make more balls to store in the freezer if you like. The tomato sauce also tastes good the way it is with pasta.

PASTA WITH AUBERGINE BALLS

SERVES 4

Tomato sauce
2 scallions (the green part)
Olive oil
2 pieces of pickled grilled pepper, plus 1 tablespoon of the oil
1 handful pitted green olives
1 can cherry tomatoes, around 1 pound (400 gram)
3 tablespoons tomato pure
1 teaspoon concentrated garlic oil or 1 teaspoon dried ramson
1–2 teaspoons sugar
1 tablespoon lemon juice
1 bay leaf
Salt
Freshly ground black pepper

Aubergine balls
2 scallions (the green part)
2 large aubergines
2 slices spelt bread or gluten-free white bread
1 handful of fresh basil
1 teaspoon dried oregano
1 handful pitted green olives
1 tablespoon lemon juice
½ tablespoon balsamic vinegar

A pinch of chili flakes
Zest of 1 lemon (save some for garnish)
Salt
Freshly ground black pepper
Olive oil
1 tablespoon basil to serve

INSTRUCTIONS

1. Make the tomato sauce: Finely chop the scallion and fry for a few minutes in some olive oil in a saucepan. Finely chop the pepper and slice the olives. Add the cherry tomatoes, tomato puree, garlic oil or ramson, peppers, olives, sugar, lemon juice, and bay leaf. Fill the empty tomato can with water and add the water to the mixture. Bring to a boil and then reduce the heat and simmer until it thickens, for about 30 to 40 minutes. Remove the bay leaf. Season to taste with salt and pepper.

2. Heat the oven to 450°F.

3. Make the aubergine balls. Finely chop the scallions and chop the aubergine into small cubes. Fry the scallion and aubergine until soft in some olive oil. Mix the bread and herbs in a food processor. Add aubergine, scallion, olives, lemon juice, balsamic vinegar, chili flakes, lemon zest, salt, and pepper. Mix in the food processor until you have a smooth batter.

4. Shape the batter into small balls. Place them on a baking pan and bake in the oven for around 20 minutes. If you use a frying pan, leave the balls to stand in the fridge for 30 minutes before you fry them. Then carefully fry them in some olive oil as they can be a bit delicate.

5. Boil the pasta according to the instructions on the packaging. Mix the pasta and tomato sauce. Add the aubergine balls, fresh basil, and some lemon zest.

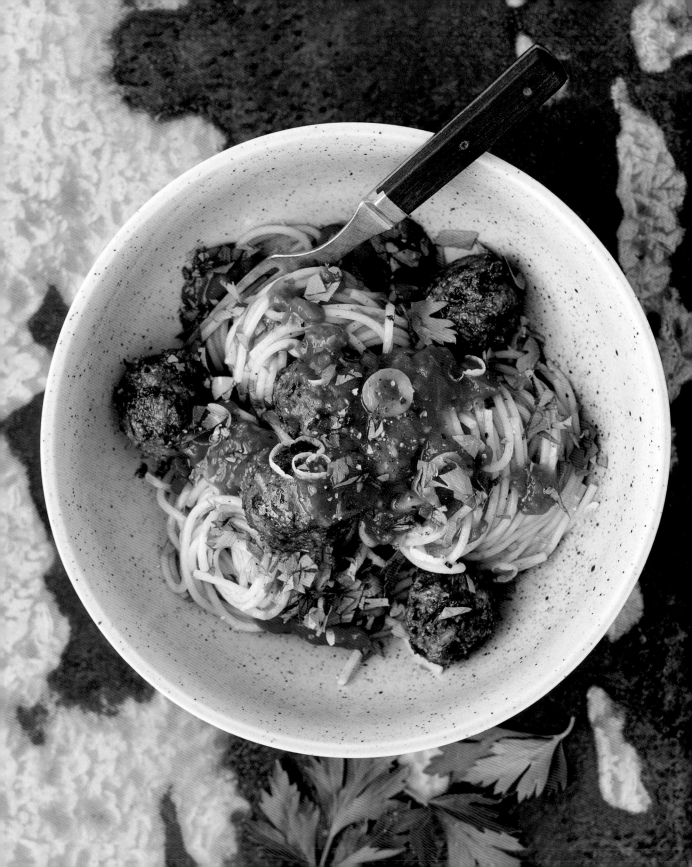

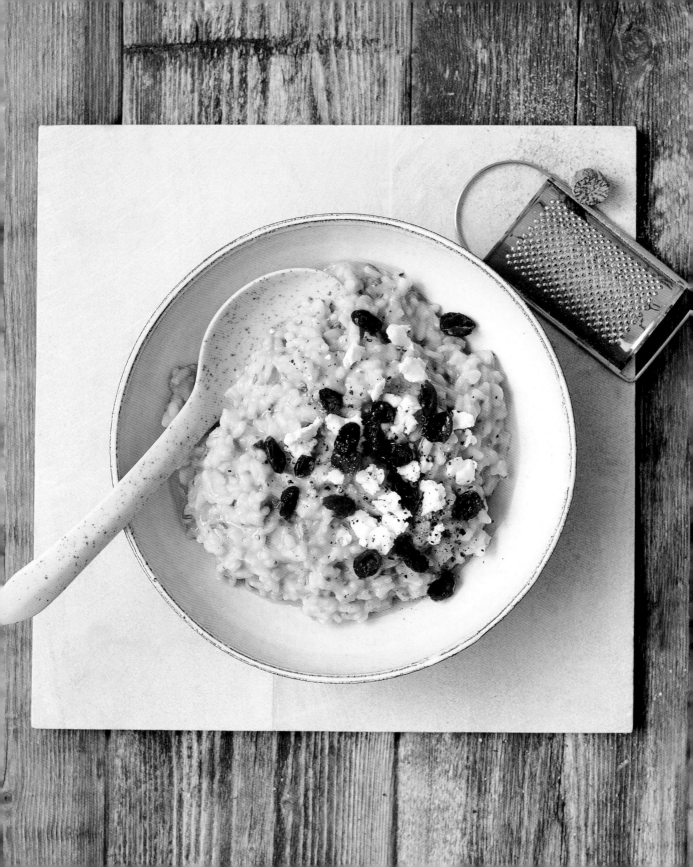

87
Pasta, risotto & stews

A delicious risotto with a salty sweet taste. Eat it as a starter, as an accompaniment to veggie burgers, or just as it is. Vegan? Replace the cheese and butter with a vegan alternative.

RISOTTO WITH SQUASH, GOAT CHEESE, AND CRANBERRIES

SERVES 4

Squash puree
2⅕ pounds squash flesh (e.g. Hokkaido)
Olive oil
Water

Risotto
2⅒ pints water
3 tablespoons onion-free vegetable stock
1 cup squash puree
2 scallions (the green part)
2 tablespoons butter
1 teaspoon salt
1 teaspoon thyme, chopped
1½ cup arborio rice
1 teaspoon white wine vinegar
⅗ cup vegetarian Parmesan, grated
⅕ cup flat leaf parsley, chopped
1 pinch nutmeg
Freshly ground black pepper
⅖ cup goat cheese, crumbled (where the lactose content is max 1g/100 g)
⅕ cup dried cranberries

INSTRUCTIONS

1. Cut the squash flesh into small pieces (Hokkaido squash does not need to be peeled). Fry in some olive oil in a saucepan. Add water so it almost covers the squash and leave to simmer under a lid for 20 minutes. Drain off the liquid, keeping it. Mix the squash to a puree and add some of the liquid from the pan until it reaches a good consistency.
2. Mix water, vegetable stock, and the squash puree in a saucepan. Reduce the heat and keep warm.
3. Finely chop and fry the scallions for a few moments in some butter. Add salt, thyme, and rice, and fry for another minute or so. Add the white wine vinegar and a ladle of the squash stock. Simmer while stirring until the liquid has been absorbed. Keep adding a ladle at a time, allowing the liquid to absorb each time. The risotto should be creamy but slightly al dente; it takes around 20 minutes.
4. Remove the saucepan from the heat and mix in the Parmesan, half the parsley, and nutmeg.
5. Season to taste with salt and pepper. Top off with some parsley, crumbled goat cheese, and dried cranberries. Serve immediately.

The perfect accompaniment to tofu or lentil burgers. Add vegetables such as zucchini, spinach, haricots vert, and black beans, and you have a complete meal! Vegan? Swap the cheese for a vegetarian alternative.

LEMON RISOTTO VERDE

SERVES 4

⅕ cup olive oil
Zest of ½ lemon
2¹⁄₁₀ pint water
2 tablespoons onion-free vegetable stock
2 scallions (the green parts)
Olive oil
1⁷⁄₁₀ cups arborio rice
⅘ cup dry white wine
⅖–⅘ cup vegetarian grated Parmesan
1¾ ounces arugula
Salt
Freshly ground pepper

INSTRUCTIONS

1. Mix some olive oil and lemon zest in a small bowl and leave to infuse while you make the risotto.
2. Heat water and stock in a saucepan. Fry the scallions until soft in some olive oil in a thick-bottomed saucepan. Fry on low heat so it doesn't catch. Add the rice and increase the heat, frying for a minute or so. Pour over the wine and cool it until the wine has evaporated, stirring the whole time.
3. Add the warm stock, a little at a time, starting with 1¼ to 1⁷⁄₁₀ cups and then ⅖ cup at a time, as the rice absorbs the stock. Keep stirring and reduce the heat. The risotto should be loose and slightly al dente. It takes around 20 minutes.
4. Remove the pan from the heat and stir in the Parmesan. Season with salt and pepper to taste. Cut the arugula into smaller pieces (save some to garnish with). Fold the arugula into the risotto. Divide the risotto between the plates and spoon over some of the lemon olive oil and garnish with arugula and vegetarian Parmesan.

TIPS

Arborio rice has a slightly higher starch content than avorio rice, but both can be used for risotto.

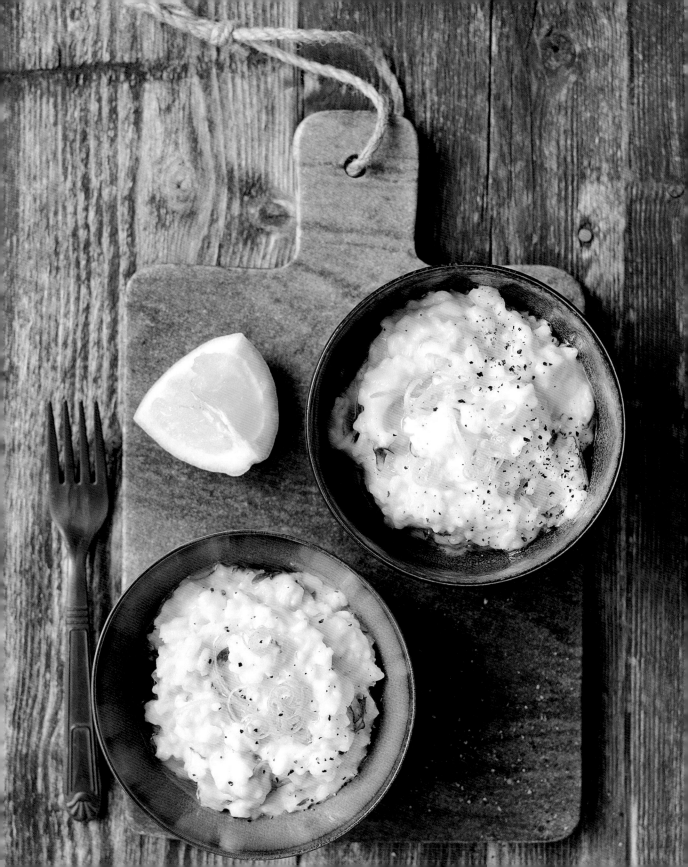

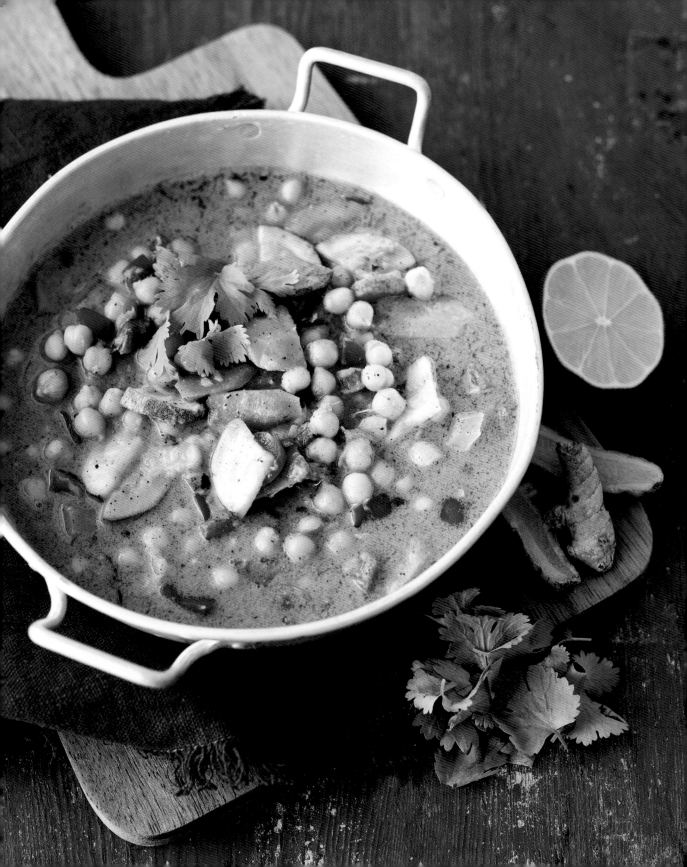

Don't let the ingredients scare you away. This is a great curry that tastes just like a curry should!

BUTTER CURRY WITH CHICKPEAS

Ⓥ

SERVES 4

3 scallions (the green part)
2⅓ inches ginger
1 teaspoon dried ramson
1 teaspoon concentrated garlic oil (optional)
2 tablespoons water
1 teaspoon ground cumin
1½ teaspoon ground coriander
½ teaspoon ground cinnamon
½ teaspoon ground cardamom
½ teaspoon cayenne pepper
Canola oil
1 teaspoon turmeric
3 tablespoons peanut butter
1⁷⁄₁₀ cups coconut milk
⅗ cup water
2 tablespoons onion-free vegetable stock
1 red pepper
2 carrots
½ zucchini
1 packet of chickpeas, ⅘ pound (380 gram)
1 teaspoon salt
1 teaspoon sugar
Juice of 1 lime
1 bunch of coriander, chopped
Chili flakes

INSTRUCTIONS

1. Mix scallions, ginger, ramson, 1 teaspoon garlic oil, and water to make a smooth puree. Fry the cumin, coriander, cinnamon, cardamom, and cayenne pepper in canola oil for around 30 seconds in a casserole or deep frying pan. Add the onion puree and stir. Mix in the turmeric and fry until the mixture is nicely brown, for around 3 minutes, stirring now and again.

2. Add peanut butter and pour in the coconut milk, water, and stock. Mix until everything has dissolved.

3. Deseed and chop the pepper and peel and chop the carrots. Cut the zucchini into half-moon shapes. Add the vegetables, drained chickpeas, salt, and sugar. Stir, place a lid on top, and leave to lightly boil for 5 minutes. Reduce the heat and leave to simmer for a further 5 minutes.

4. Add lime juice and coriander and add chili flakes to taste. Keep simmering for another 3 to 4 minutes until the curry thickens.

5. Eat it as is, or serve with rice or bread.

A child-friendly meal that hides lots of vegetables and lentils without anyone noticing. It has a lovely taste of curry and coconut. This dish can also be frozen.

92

Pasta, risotto & stews

AUBERGINE AND LENTIL CURRY

SERVES 4

2 scallions (the green part)
1 large or 2 small aubergines
2 carrots
Olive oil
2 teaspoons curry
2 teaspoons ground ginger
2 teaspoons ground coriander
2 teaspoons turmeric
1 can coconut milk, ⅘ pints (400 ml)
1 can crushed tomatoes, ½ pound
1-2 tablespoons onion-free vegetable stock
⅔ cup water
⅘ cup of green lentils from a carton
Salt
Some cayenne pepper

INSTRUCTIONS

1. Finely chop the scallions and dice the aubergine into small pieces. Peel and dice the carrots. Fry the aubergine, carrots, and scallions in oil for around 5 minutes, stirring occasionally.

2. Dust some curry, ginger, coriander, and turmeric on top. Add coconut milk, crushed tomatoes, stock, and water. Leave to simmer for 10 minutes. Rinse the lentils and add them to the pot. Season to taste with salt and cayenne pepper.

3. Serve the curry with rice, barley, or quinoa.

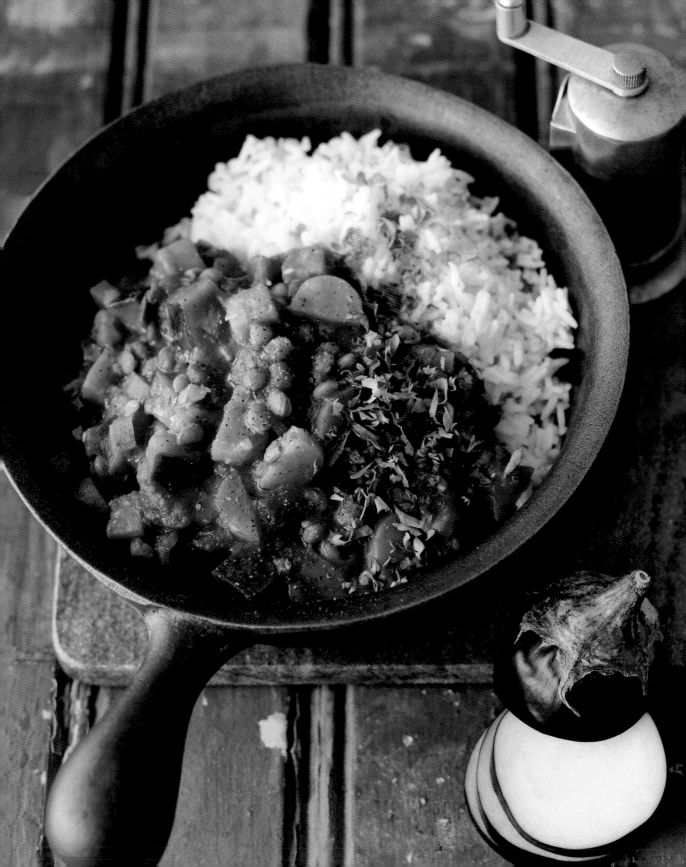

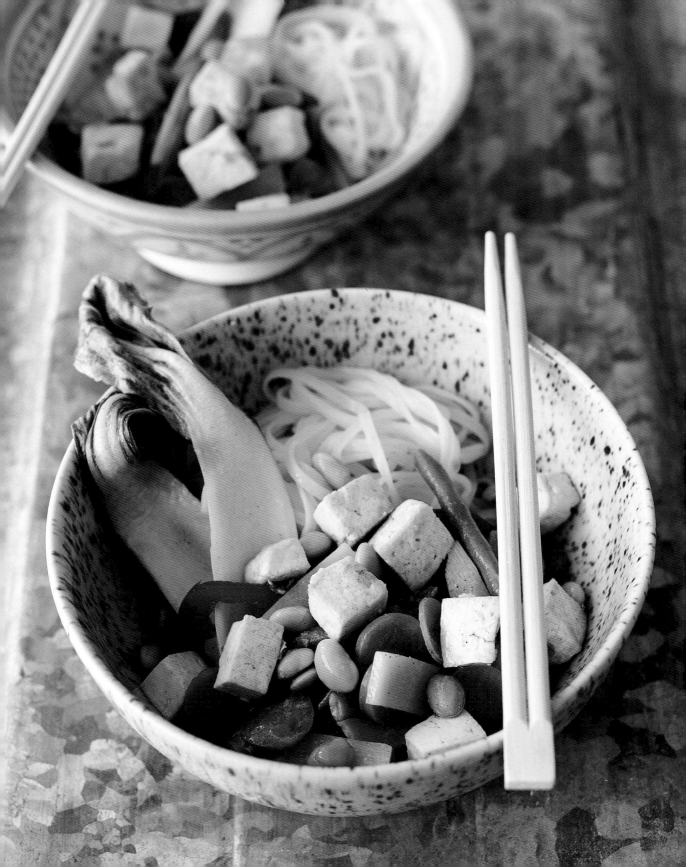

*It's almost impossible to find curry paste without
garlic, so you most likely will have to make your own.
Whatever is left can be kept in the fridge and used in
other dishes.*

TOFU WOK WITH GREEN CURRY

SERVES 4

Curry paste
5 scallions (the green part)
½ bunch coriander
2 green chilies, seeds removed
2 stalks lemongrass (remove the
    outer leaves and slice the rest)
6 inches ginger, peeled
1 tablespoon fish sauce

Tofu
½ pound natural tofu
2 tablespoons canola oil
Chili oil or chili flakes
Salt

Curry
1 red bell pepper
1 carrot
3½ ounces haricots vert

½ pound bok choy
2 tablespoons oil, preferably
    flavored with garlic
1 can bamboo shoots, about
    ½ pound (230 gram)
⅔ cup edamame
6 kaffir lime leaves
1 can coconut milk,
    ⅘ pints (400 ml)
Juice of ½ lime

INSTRUCTIONS

1. Mix all the ingredients for the
   curry paste into a smooth paste
   in a food processor or with a
   stick blender.
2. Cut the tofu into smaller cubes.
   Heat some canola oil and chili
   oil or chili flakes in a large

frying pan and fry the tofu until
golden brown. Lightly salt and
place the tofu on a plate.

3. Deseed the pepper and slice
   thinly and peel and thinly slice
   the carrot. Divide the haricots
   vert down the middle and
   remove the leaves on the bok
   choy. Heat the oil in a large
   frying pan and fry the curry
   paste on medium heat for a
   minute or so. Add pepper,
   carrot, haricots vert, bok choy,
   bamboo shoots, edamame, and
   kaffir lime leaves.
4. Add the coconut milk and tofu
   and leave to simmer for 10 to
   15 minutes. Add lime juice to
   taste. Serve the curry with rice
   noodles.

This is vegetable mix that tastes better the longer it cooks. Wild rice gives it a bit of bite and adds flavor. Feel free to double the recipe and freeze to eat as a side to another meal, like pasta. Vegan? Swap the halloumi for a vegan alternative.

RATATOUILLE WITH WILD RICE AND FRIED HALLOUMI

SERVES 4

1 large zucchini
1 parsnip
1 red bell pepper
1 green bell pepper
1 leek (the green part)
2 bay leaves
Olive oil
2 cans whole tomatoes, around ½ pound each (400 gram)
1 teaspoon dried oregano
1 teaspoon dried thyme
1 teaspoon dried basil
1 teaspoon dried rosemary
5 leaves freshly chopped ramson or 1 teaspoon dried
5⅓ ounces halloumi (where the lactose content is max 1g/100 g)
Juice of ½ lemon
Bunch parsley
Salt
Freshly ground pepper

INSTRUCTIONS

1. Cut the zucchini into ½ inch thick half-moon shapes. Peel and slice the parsnip into half-moon shapes. Deseed the peppers and cut into rough strips. Rinse and roughly shred the leek.
2. Fry the vegetables and the bay leaves in some oil in a casserole dish. Add the whole tomatoes, oregano, thyme, basil, rosemary, and ramson. If it looks too dry, add some water. Stir and leave to summer under a lid on low heat for around 40 minutes. Remove bay leaves.
3. Slice the halloumi and fry until golden brown in a dry frying pan. Add lemon juice, salt, and pepper to taste to the ratatouille. Chop lots of fresh parsley over it and serve with the halloumi and wild rice.

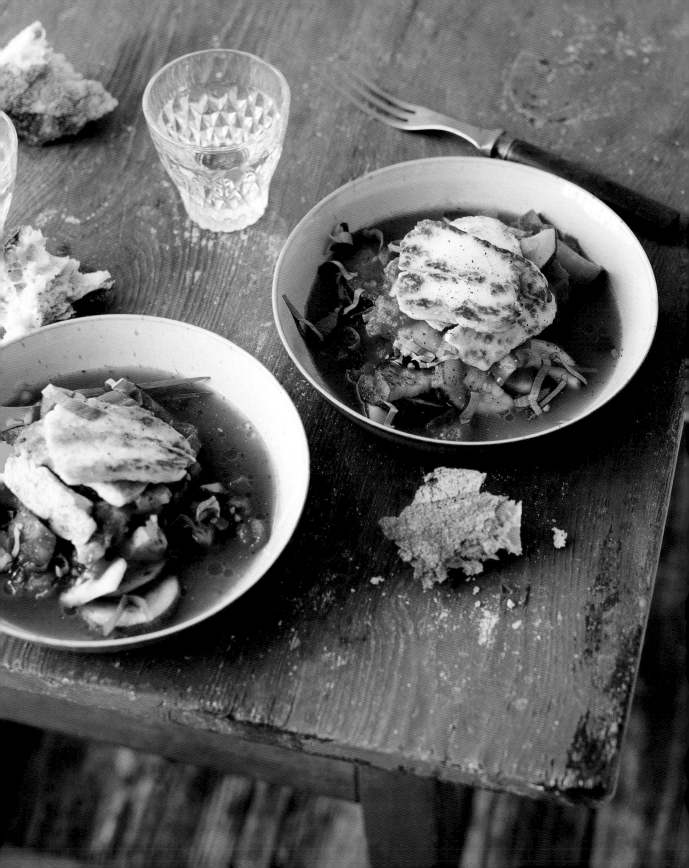

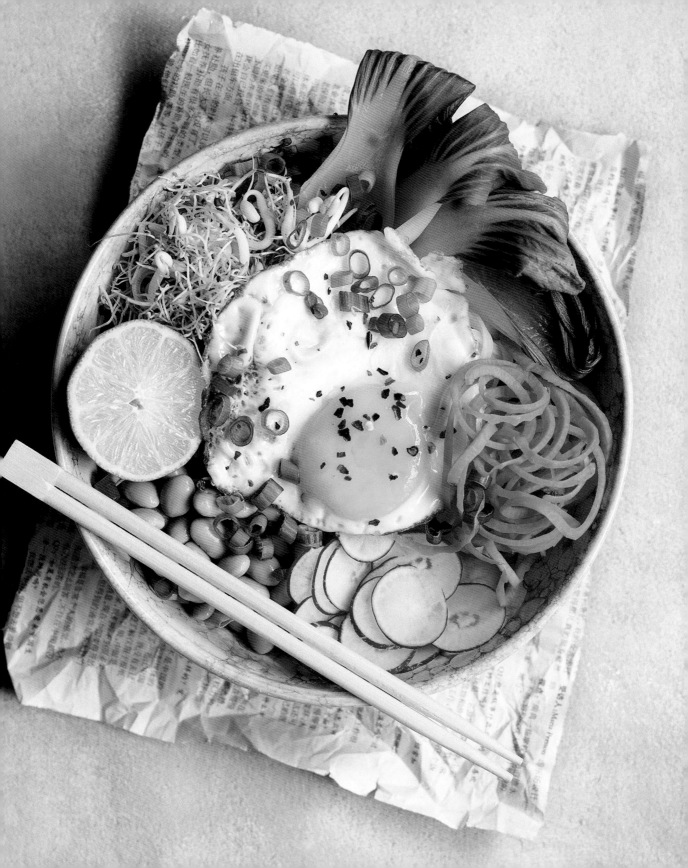

A fast weekday dish where you can use vegetables you already have at home. Vegan? Skip the egg and add some tofu instead if you like.

VEGGIE BOWL

SERVES 4

2 garlic cloves
2 scallions (the green part)
1⅗ inches fresh ginger
Olive oil
1 red chili
2½ pints water
2½ teaspoons onion-free vegetable stock
2 tablespoons tamari
1 tablespoon syrup
1½ tablespoons white wine vinegar
2 carrots
½ pound bok choy
12 radishes
1½ tablespoons sesame oil
7 ounces rice noodles
4 eggs
1 carton bean sprouts
⅖ cup edamame
1 lime
Chili flakes

INSTRUCTIONS

1. Peel and chop the garlic into pieces. Finely chop the scallions and grate the ginger. Fry the garlic in oil until it catches color. Remove the garlic (make sure you remove all of it) and discard. Place the scallion, chili, and ginger in the oil and fry for about 1 minute. Add water, vegetable stock, tamari, syrup, and white wine vinegar and simmer for 20 minutes.

2. Peel and cut the carrots into small sticks or shave with a potato peeler. Roughly chop the bok choy and thinly slice the radishes. Place the radishes to one side. Add carrots, bok choy, and sesame oil and simmer for a further 5 minutes. Cook the noodles according to the instructions on the packaging and rinse them in cold water. Fry the eggs on one side.

3. Place the noodles in a bowl. Add bean sprouts, edamame, and radishes, and then pour over the warm stock with carrot and bok choy. Top off with eggs, a wedge of lime, and chili flakes.

TIPS

Edamame can be found whole or shelled in the freezer section.

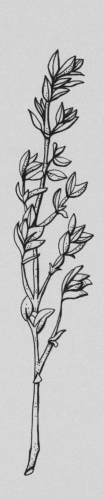

Pies, wraps & burgers

Pie is perfect to freeze and take to work for lunch. You can replace sorghum and cornmeal with sieved spelt flour.

102
*Pies, wraps
& burgers*

GOAT CHEESE AND BASIL PIE

SERVES 4 TO 6

Piecrust
⅗ cup sorghum flour
⅗ cup cornmeal
1 teaspoon baking powder
1¾ ounce butter at room
    temperature
⅖ cup lactose-free milk

Filling
½ pound fresh or frozen broccoli
8 sun-dried tomatoes
5⅓ ounces fresh spinach
Butter
3 tablespoons pine nuts
3 eggs
1¼ cups lactose-free cream for
    cooking or milk
Salt
Freshly ground pepper
1 bunch chopped basil
4⅖ ounces goat cheese (where
    the amount of lactose is max
    1g/100 g)

INSTRUCTIONS

1. Heat the oven to 400°F. Mix all the ingredients for the piecrust and press into a pie pan. Lightly prick with a fork and blind bake the crust in the oven for 10 to 15 minutes.

2. Cut the broccoli and tomatoes into pieces. Fry the spinach with some butter in a frying pan. Roast the pine nuts in a dry frying pan. Whisk together the eggs, cream, salt, and pepper. Place the spinach, broccoli, basil, sun-dried tomatoes, and pine nuts in the piecrust and pour over the egg mixture. Slice the goat cheese and place on top of the pie.

3. Bake in the middle of the oven for around 20 minutes until the cheese has turned a nice color. Serve with a green salad.

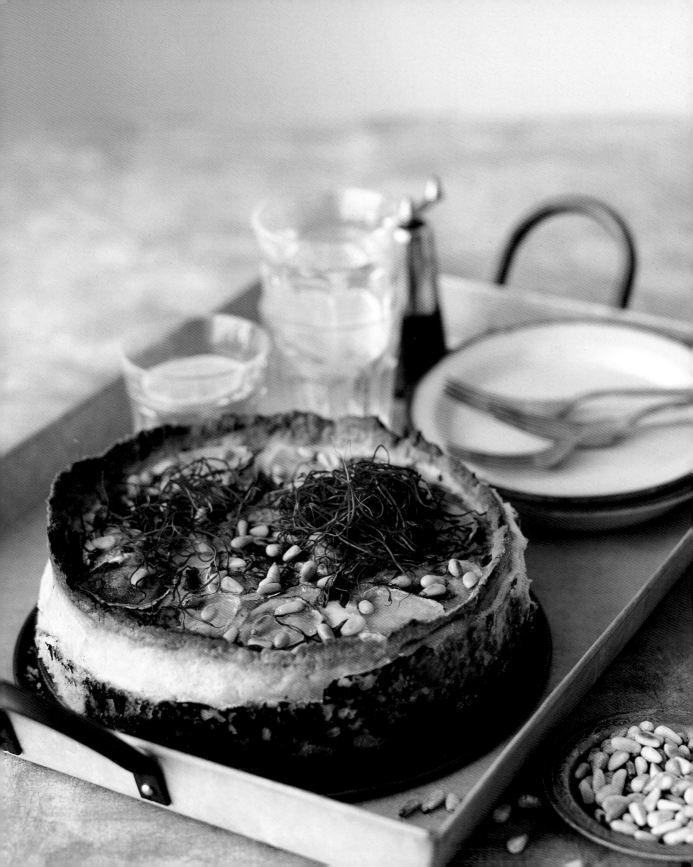

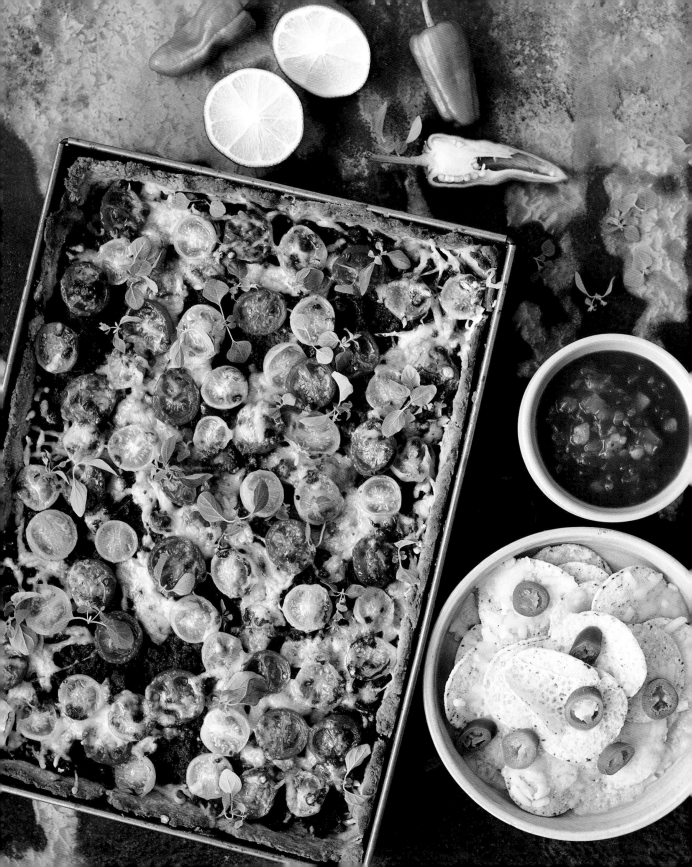

This is new twist on the regular Taco Tuesday. Make double the amount of salsa and keep in the fridge. There is onion-free taco seasoning to buy or you can easily make your own. Vegan? Use a dairy-free margarine, oat fraîche, and vegan cheese.

TACO PIE WITH QUORN

SERVES 4 TO 6

Piecrust
1¼ cup gluten-free flour mix or sieved spelt flour
1 pinch salt
2⅗ ounces butter
⅖ cup lactose-free quark
2 tablespoons water

Salsa
1 can chopped tomatoes
4 sun-dried tomatoes
7 sprigs oregano
5 sprigs thyme
20 basil leaves
½ tablespoon brown sugar
Salt
Freshly ground black pepper
1 teaspoon concentrated garlic oil (optional)
1 red chili pepper (depending on desired strength)
½ fresh pineapple or one small can

Filling
1 pound Quorn Grounds
Butter
3–4 teaspoons onion-free taco seasoning
⅖ cup water
⅖ cup lactose-free crème fraîche
2 cartons of cocktail tomatoes
⅘–1¼ cups grated cheese
Butter

INSTRUCTIONS

1. Mix flour, salt, and finely cubed butter for the piecrust with your hands or in a food processor. Add quark and water and mix together to make a smooth dough. Leave to rest in the fridge for an hour.
2. Heat the oven to 450°F.
3. Press the dough into a pie pan and prick with a fork. Blind bake in the middle of the oven for around 10 minutes.
4. Pour the chopped tomatoes into a saucepan. Finely chop the sun-dried tomatoes and herbs and stir into the pan. Add brown sugar, salt, pepper, garlic oil, and finely chopped chili. Leave to simmer on low heat for 20 minutes until everything is combined. Pour into a bowl and leave to cool.
5. Peel the pineapple and remove the hard core. Cut into cubes and stir into the tomato sauce.
6. Brown the Quorn Grounds in a frying pan with some butter. Add the taco seasoning and water. Leave to simmer for 10 to 15 minutes. Stir in the crème fraîche and mix thoroughly. Fill the piecrust with the Quorn Grounds. Halve the tomatoes and place on top. Add the cheese and bake the pie in the middle of the oven for 20 to 30 minutes.
7. Serve with a green salad, tomatoes, cucumber, pineapple salsa, and tortilla chips.

Mix in some chopped herbs such as parsley and oregano to give it a slightly more exciting taste. If you are not eating the tortillas straight away you can store them in a plastic bag for a few days and then warm them in the oven. They can also be frozen.

TIPS

More wholemeal means more FODMAP. That's why wholemeal spelt is not allowed.

SPELT TORTILLA

MAKES 8

2½ cups sieved spelt flour
1 teaspoon baking powder
1 teaspoon salt
⅘ cup cold water
2 tablespoons olive oil

INSTRUCTIONS

1. Mix the flour, baking powder, and salt in a bowl. Add water and oil and work into a smooth dough. Divide the dough into 8 equal-size pieces and flatten them into rounds on a lightly floured surface. Roll them out thinly, at around 1 to 2 mm thick.

2. Fry the tortillas in a hot, dry frying pan for around 1 minute per side. They should get some color, but not become too hard, as they can be harder to roll and become dry. Leave them to cool down under a towel.

SPELT BREAD

MAKES 3

1¾ ounces yeast
5½ cups water at 98.6°F
1¾ ounces butter at room
    temperature
2 teaspoons salt
2⅕ cups sieved spelt flour, divided

INSTRUCTIONS

1. Crumble the yeast into a large bowl. Pour over the water and stir until the yeast dissolves. Add butter, salt, and 2 cups flour (save ⅕ cup for rolling out the dough). Knead the dough thoroughly until it is smooth, around 5 minutes in a food processor, or with an electric whisk with a dough hook. Prove until it doubles in size under a towel, around 30 minutes.
2. Turn out the dough on a floured surface and lightly knead. Divide into three parts and shape into round loaves. Place the bread on a sheet pan lined with parchment paper or in greased loaf pans (3⅕ pints). Proof under a towel for 40 minutes.
3. Heat the oven to 450°F. Brush the loaves with some water and score with a sharp knife.
4. Bake in the lower part of the oven for around 25 minutes. Leave to cool on a baking rack without a towel to give it a crispy crust.

CORN TORTILLA

MAKES 10

1⁷⁄₁₀ cups water
1 cup corn flour
⅖ cup corn starch
1½ teaspoons baking powder
3 tablespoons fibre husk
1 teaspoon salt

INSTRUCTIONS

1. Mix all the ingredients to make a dough and leave to swell for 20 minutes. Divide the dough into 10 bits on a lightly floured surface and roll them out to 2 mm-thick round breads.
2. Fry on high heat in a dry frying pan. Fry each side for a few minutes until they turn a nice color. Place the finished tortillas in a towel or keep them warm in the oven until it's time to eat.

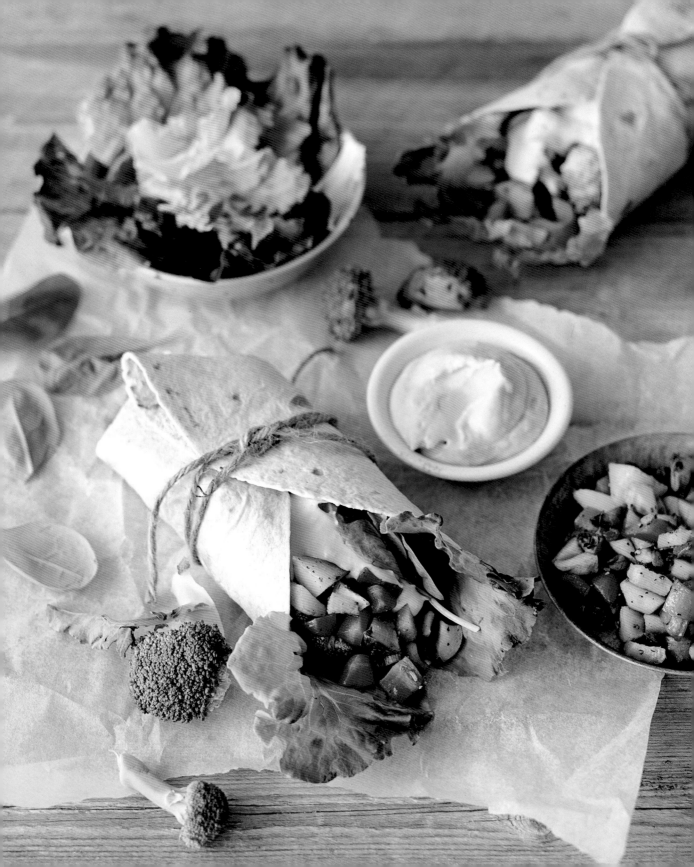

Fill the wrap with whatever you have at home. Leftovers work well for this—leftovers from the root vegetable hash would be good. Barley is also good to use as a filling. Hummus can be made in a big batch and kept in the fridge. It's nice as a dip or on a sandwich. Vegan? Replace the cheese with a vegan alternative.

GREEN WRAP WITH HUMMUS

MAKES 4

1 carton chickpeas, ⅘ pound (380 gram)

3 tablespoons olive oil

2 teaspoons concentrated garlic oil

2 tablespoons tahini (sesame seed paste)

½ tablespoon lemon juice

1 teaspoon ground cumin

Salt

Freshly ground black pepper

2½ ounces fresh spinach

4⅖ ounces frozen broccoli

4 tortilla breads, such as spelt or corn (see previous page)

A few slices sharp cheese

INSTRUCTIONS

1. Drain and rinse the chickpeas and mix them together with the olive oil. Add garlic oil, tahini, lemon juice, and cumin. Season to taste with salt and pepper.
2. Rinse the spinach. Defrost the broccoli and cut into small pieces.
3. Place the spinach, broccoli, and hummus on the tortilla breads. If you like you can add root vegetables or barley. Top off with a few slices of sharp cheese and fold.

Aivar relish is a mixture based on peppers. There are varieties without garlic, but you can easily make your own. Vegan? Use oat fraîche and replace the halloumi with a vegan alternative.

HALLUMI WRAP WITH AIVAR

MAKES 4

½ aubergine
1 red chili
3 tablespoons olive oil
1½ pickled pepper
Salt
1½ cups lactose-free crème fraîche
Freshly ground black pepper
5⅓ ounces halloumi
1 bell pepper (any color)
1 zucchini
Lettuce leaves
4 tortillas, e.g. spelt or corn
   (see page 106-107)

INSTRUCTIONS

1. Heat the oven to 400°F. Halve the ½ of aubergine lengthwise and place it with the chili in an oven proof dish with a little olive oil. Roast in the oven for 20 to 25 minutes.
2. Cube the pepper. Mix peppers, eggplant (skin on), chili, salt, and olive oil in a food processor or with a stick blender until smooth.
3. Mix the pepper mixture, crème fraîche, salt, and pepper. Place the aivar sauce in a cold place.

Slice the halloumi and dry fry in a frying pan. Shred the fresh pepper and shave strips of zucchini with a mandoline or cheese slicer. Place the halloumi, bell pepper, zucchini, and lettuce and aivar sauce on the tortillas and fold.

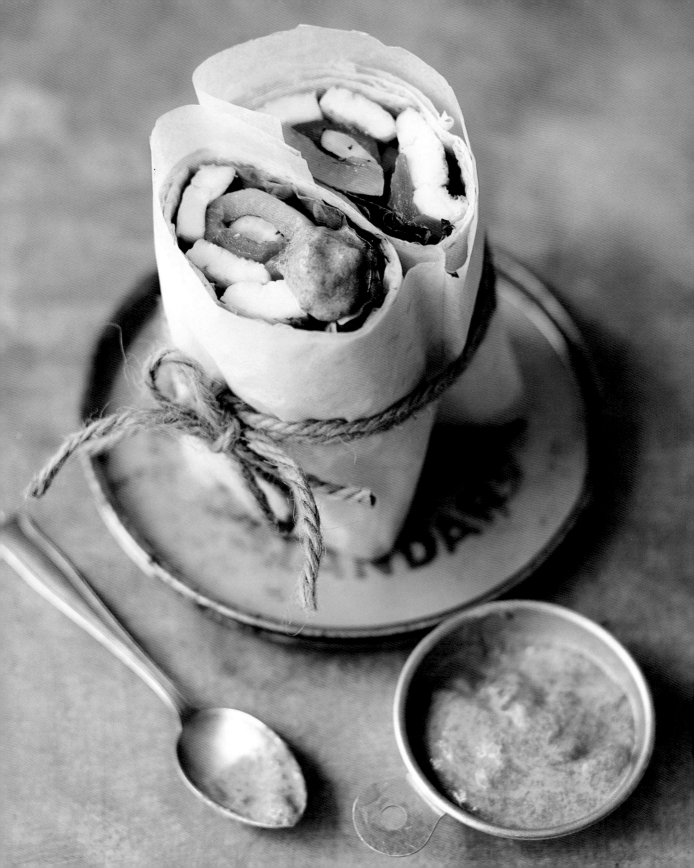

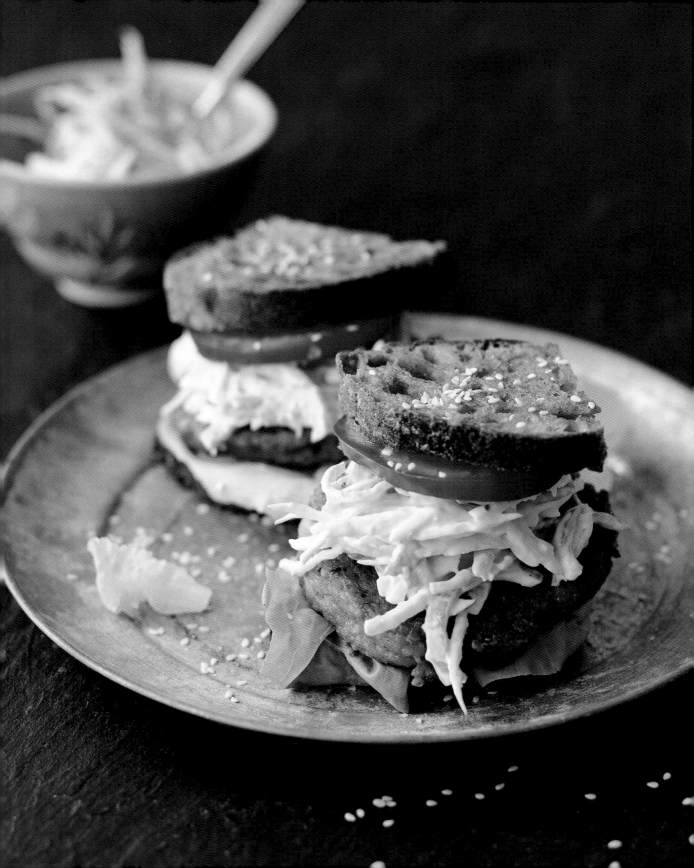

Vegan? Replace the mozzarella with a vegan alternative, replace the eggs with 1 tablespoon potato flour, skip the mayonnaise, and use oat fraîche.

QUINOA BURGERS WITH COLESLAW

SERVES 4

Burgers
1 cup red quinoa
Olive oil
2¹⁄₁₀ cups water
1½ tablespoons onion-free
   vegetable stock
4²⁄₅ grams mozzarella
2 scallions (the green parts)
4 sun-dried tomatoes
2 eggs
3 tablespoons sieved spelt flour
1 teaspoon ramson
Salt
Freshly ground black pepper
Canola oil

Coleslaw
⅓ cup mayonnaise
3 tablespoons lactose-free Greek
   yogurt
1 teaspoon Dijon mustard
A few splashes of Tabasco

⅗ pound pointed cabbage
1 carrot
2 inches finely shredded leek
   (the green part)
½ fresh parsley, finely chopped

To serve
4 slices bread, such as spelt bread
   (see recipe on page 107)
A few lettuce leaves
Olive oil
Sliced tomato

INSTRUCTIONS

1. Rinse the quinoa and fry in
   some olive oil for 2 minutes.
   Add water and stock. Mix and
   bring to a boil. Reduce the heat
   and simmer under a lid for 15
   minutes.
2. Coleslaw: Mix mayonnaise,
   yogurt, Dijon mustard, and

Tabasco in a large bowl.
Shred the pointed cabbage
and roughly grate the carrot.
Add the cabbage, carrot, leek
and parsley, folding it into the
mixture.
3. Finely chop mozzarella, scallions,
   and tomatoes. Whisk the eggs,
   and mix with the quinoa and the
   rest of the ingredients to make a
   batter. Shape into 4 burgers. Add
   some more spelt if the batter is
   too loose. Heat some canola oil
   in a frying pan. Fry the burgers
   for a few minutes on each side
   until they turn golden brown.
   Place them to cool on some
   kitchen towel.
4. Fry the bread slices in a hot
   frying pan with some olive oil.
   Divide down the middle and
   make burgers from the quinoa
   burgers, lettuce leaves, and
   tomatoes.

Vegan? Replace the halloumi with a vegetarian alternative.

114
*Pies, wraps
& burgers*

LENTIL AND CHICKPEA BURGERS WITH CUCUMBER SALAD

SERVES 4

Burgers
1 carton chickpeas, ⅖ pound
    (190 grams)
1 carton red lentils, ⅘ pound
    (380 grams)
1½ cups thawed spinach leaves
1 teaspoon ancho chili powder
1 teaspoon ground cumin
⅕ cup corn starch
Salt
Freshly ground black pepper
2⅗ ounces halloumi (where
    the lactose content is max
    1g/100 g)
⅖ cup sunflower seeds, roasted
    and unsalted
1 bunch coriander

Cucumber salad
2 cucumbers
1 teaspoon salt
2 carrots
1 red bell pepper
2 tablespoons finely chopped
    fresh cilantro
1 tablespoon sesame seeds, white
    or black

Dressing
2 tablespoons rice vinegar
Juice of ½ lemon
1 tablespoon soy sauce
1 tablespoon maple syrup
1 teaspoon ginger, grated
1 tablespoon sesame oil

Millet
1 cup millet
1 tablespoon olive oil
1⁷⁄₁₀ cups hot water
½ gram saffron
Salt

INSTRUCTIONS

1. Drain and rinse the chickpeas.
   Squeeze the liquid from the
   spinach. Mix the chickpeas,
   lentils, spinach, ancho chili,
   cumin, corn starch, salt,
   and black pepper in a food
   processor or with a stick
   blender to make a smooth
   mixture. Grate the halloumi.
   Add the halloumi, sunflower
   seeds, and finely chopped
   coriander into the mixture.
   Make 4 burgers with oiled
   hands. Grill or fry the burgers
   for 3 to 4 minutes on each side.
2. Halve the cucumbers
   lengthways, remove the seeds,
   and shave into strips. Place in a
   colander and mix with the salt.
   Leave to sweat out the water
   for around 15 minutes.
3. Peel and shave the carrots in
   the same way. Cut the peppers
   into thin strips. Place the
   cucumber on a kitchen towel
   and remove as much moisture
   as possible.
4. Mix all the ingredients for the
   dressing and add the cucumber,
   carrots, and peppers. Top off
   with chopped coriander and
   sesame seeds.
5. Rinse the millet in cold water
   and then boiling water. Fry
   in some olive oil for a minute
   or so. Add water, saffron, and
   salt, and cook according to the
   instructions. Leave to cool.
   Serve with the burgers and
   cucumber salad.

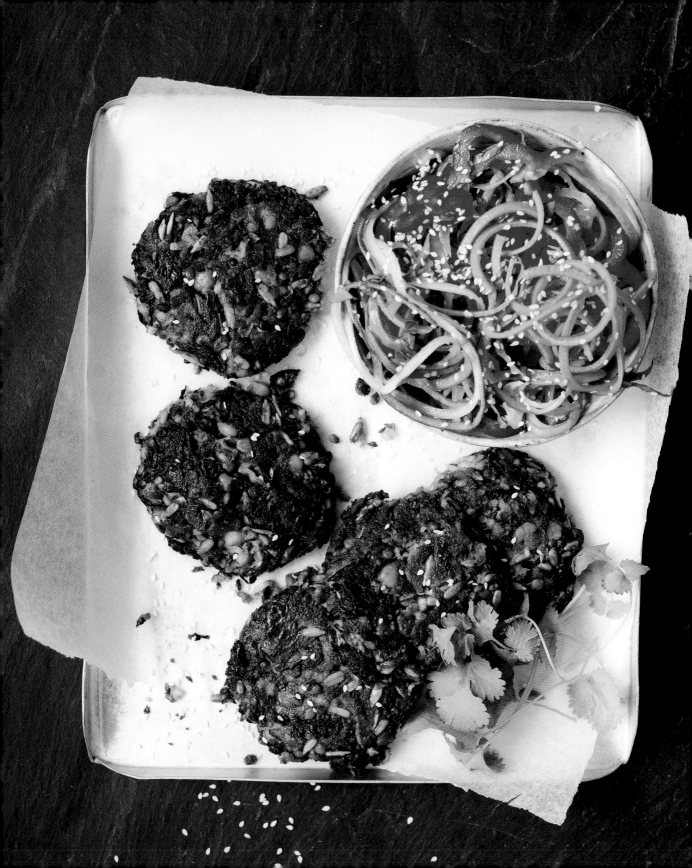

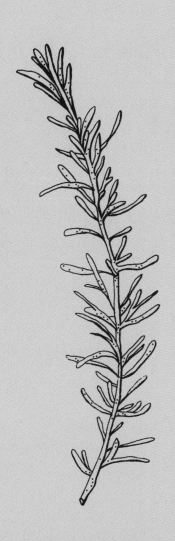

Home cooking & finger food

There's a Swedish saying, "use what you already have," and that is just what this dish is all about—using the vegetables you have at home. Pickled beets can be eaten as they are fermented, and so gentle on the gut. Vegan? Skip the eggs.

VEGETABLE HASH WITH PICKLED BEETS AND EGGS

SERVES 4

2 scallions (the green part)
8 potatoes
4 parsnips
½ celeriac
2 large carrots
Olive oil
Salt
Freshly ground pepper
1 teaspoon thyme
1 teaspoon rosemary

To serve
Fried eggs
Pickled beets

INSTRUCTIONS

1. Heat the oven to 425°F. Finely chop the scallions. Peel and chop the potatoes and root vegetables into ½-inch cubes. Place on a pan and drizzle over some olive oil. Add salt and pepper. Add some thyme and rosemary and give it a good stir.

2. Bake in the middle of the oven for 20 to 25 minutes, stirring now and again. Serve the hash with fried eggs and pickled beets.

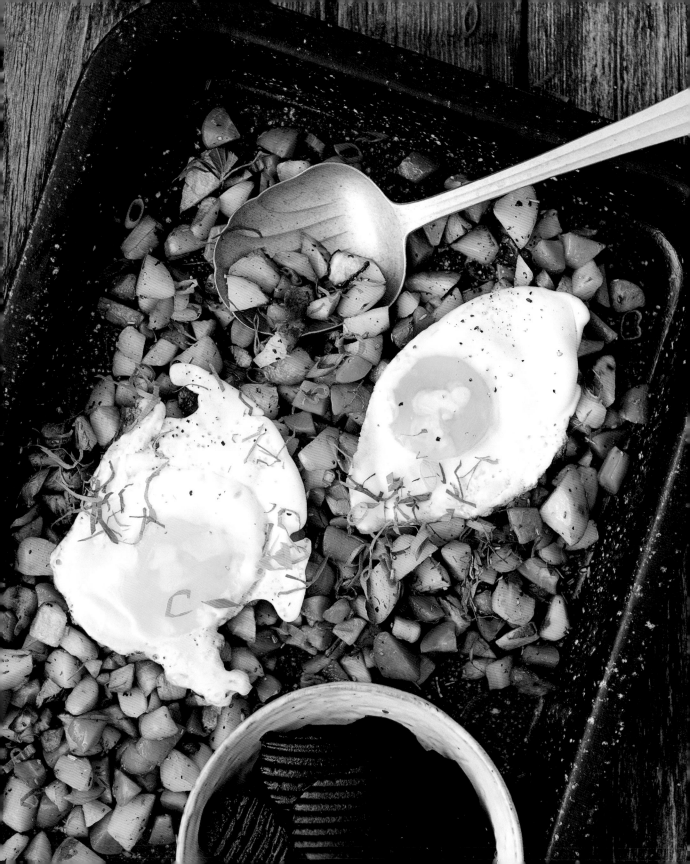

Vegan? Use dairy-free margarine and oat milk or rice milk and rice cream.

120
Home cooking & finger food

QUORN PARCELS

SERVES 4

Quorn parcels
1 white cabbage
1⅓ pounds Quorn
⅓ cup cooked rice
⅘ cup lactose-free milk
2 eggs
1 teaspoon soy sauce
2 teaspoons ground cinnamon
1½ tablespoons onion-free
    vegetable stock
2 tablespoons melted butter
2 tablespoons light syrup
⅘ cup water
Butter for greasing
Salt
Freshly ground black pepper

Cream sauce
⅖ cup jus from the pan
⅖ cup brine from the cabbage
⅘ cup lactose-free cream for
    cooking
½ tablespoon soya sauce
½ tablespoon balsamic vinegar
½ tablespoon vegetable stock

Pressed cucumber
1 fresh cucumber
2 tablespoons white vinegar (12%)
⅖ cup water

2 tablespoons sugar
½ pinch ground white pepper
2 tablespoons chopped parsley

Lingonberries
¼ pound frozen lingonberries
⅖ cups sugar

To serve
Boiled or mashed potatoes

INSTRUCTIONS

1. Start with the pressed
   cucumber. Thinly slice the
   cucumber. Make a brine from
   the vinegar, water, sugar, white
   pepper, and parsley. Mix until
   the sugar dissolves. Place the
   cucumber in a jar and pour over
   the brine. Leave for an hour or
   so before serving.
2. Mix the lingonberries and sugar
   and set aside until ready to
   serve.
3. Cut the base off the cabbage
   and parboil in lightly salted
   water for around 15 minutes.
   Remove with a skimmer and
   carefully loosen the leaves.
   Remove the hard middle

sections. Save ⅘ cups of the
water from boiling. Place the
leaves on a chopping board.

4. Heat the oven to 400°F. Mix
   the Quorn, rice, milk, eggs, soy
   sauce, cinnamon, and stock.
   Add salt and pepper. Place in a
   food processor and blend until
   smooth. Dollop the mixture
   onto the cabbage leaves and
   roll them into tight parcels and
   place in a greased, oven-safe
   dish. Brush the parcels with
   melted butter and syrup.
5. Bake in the middle of the oven
   for around 30 minutes until the
   parcels have caught a nice color.
   Add ⅘ cups water to the pan
   and lower the heat to 300°F.
   Cook for an additional 30 to 40
   minutes and cover with jus now
   and again.
6. Whisk together the ingredients
   for the sauce in a frying pan.
   Bring to a boil and add salt and
   pepper to taste.
7. Serve the Quorn parcels
   with boiled potato, cream
   sauce, pressed cucumber, and
   lingonberries.

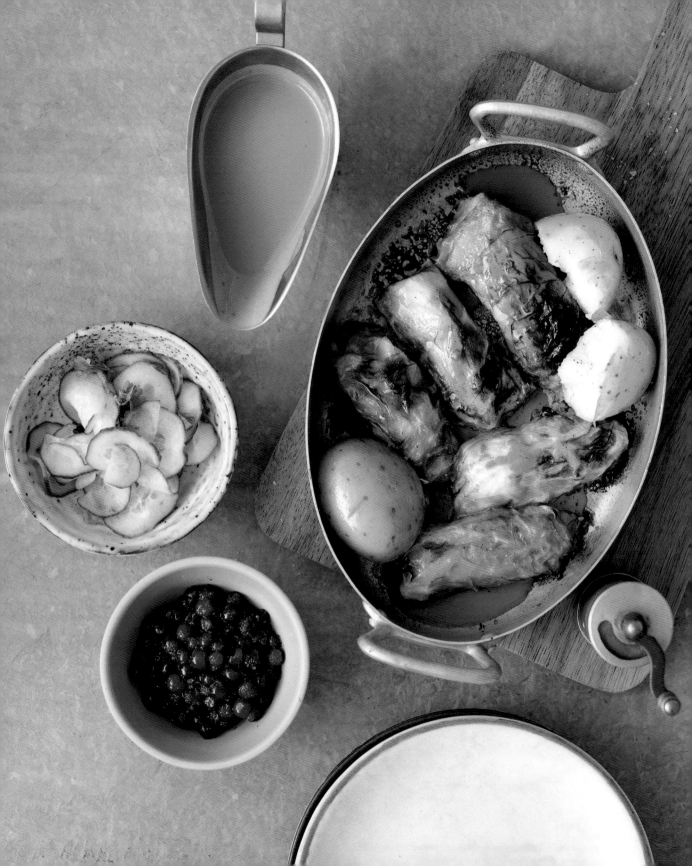

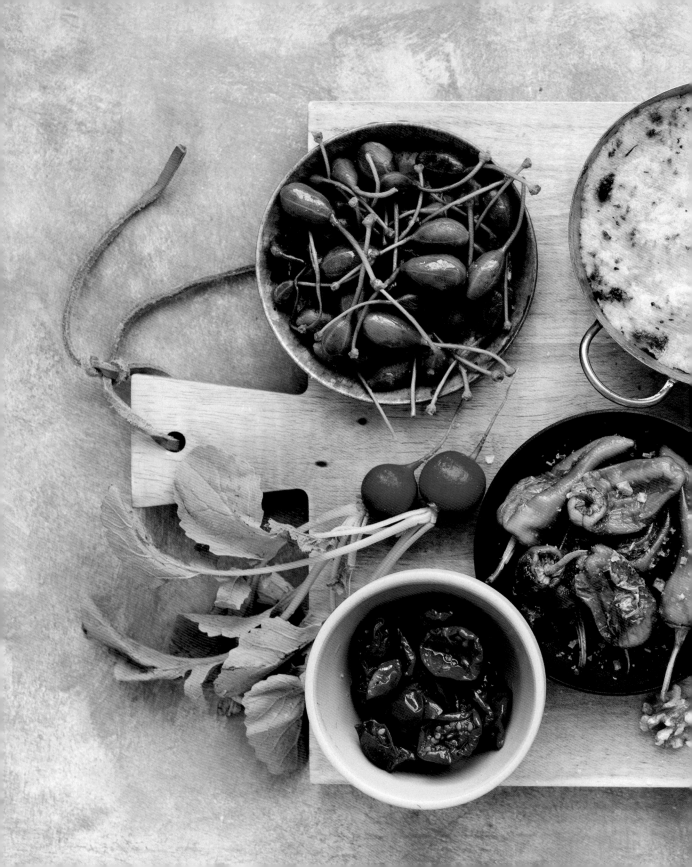

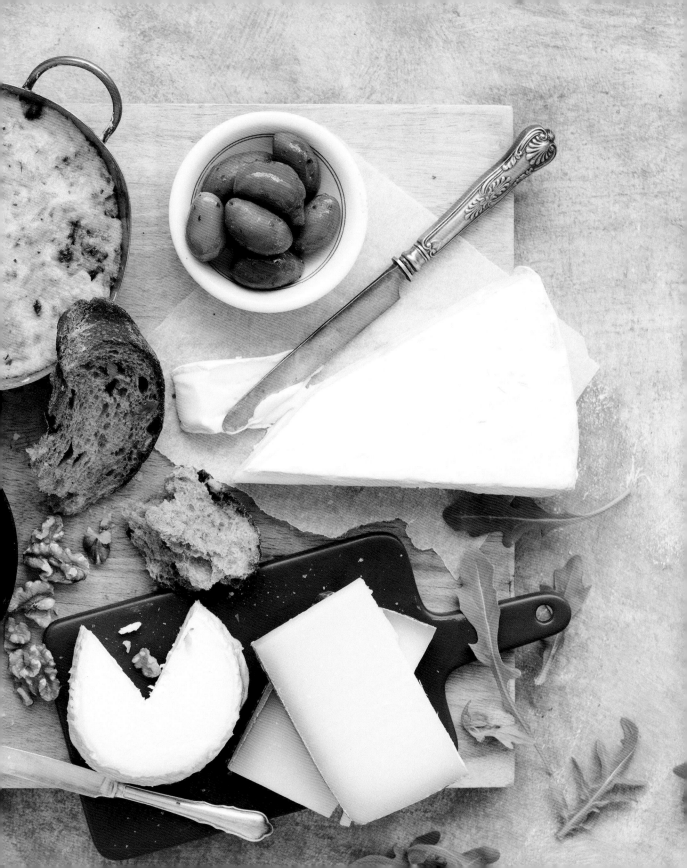

Whether you are having a big party or a staying in, finger food is perfect to serve at a dinner party, buffet, or for a cozy Friday night in.

124
Home cooking & finger food

FINGER FOOD *(see images on previous pages)*

SERVES 4

Semidried tomatoes

1. Halve cherry tomatoes and place on a sheet pan lined with parchment paper.
2. Drizzle over some olive oil, salt, and pepper.
3. Bake at 200°F for around 3 hours.

Pimientos de padron

1. Fry the pimientos (small green peppers) on medium heat in a frying pan with olive oil until they turn a nice color and are slightly reduced in size.
2. Sprinkle some flaked salt on top and serve.

Accompaniments

Capers
Radishes
Olives
Dessert cheeses
Hummus (see page 109)

*Vegan? Replace the yogurt with an oat-based
alternative.*

FINGER FOOD *(image on following page)*

SERVES 4

*Aubergine with feta cheese and
pomegranate*
2 aubergines
Olive oil
Freshly ground pepper
⅔ cup lactose-free Greek yogurt
½ bunch coriander
Juice of 1 lemon
Dried ramson (optional)
Salt
1 pomegranate
Walnuts

INSTRUCTIONS

1. Divide the aubergine
   lengthwise in ¾-inch-thick
   slices. Sprinkle over some salt
   and place in a colander. Place
   a weight on top and leave for
   around 1 hour.
2. Heat a griddle pan or normal
   frying pan to high heat. Drizzle
   olive oil over the aubergine
   slices and season with pepper.
   Grill for 3 to 4 minutes on each
   side until golden brown.
3. Mix yogurt, finely chopped
   coriander, lemon juice, ramson,
   salt and pepper in a bowl.
   Deseed the pomegranate. Top
   off the aubergines with the
   yogurt sauce, pomegranate
   seeds, and walnuts.

Oven-baked pointed cabbage
2 pointed cabbages
4 tablespoons lactose-free cream
   for cooking
Sharp cheese or vegetarian
   Parmesan
Salt
Freshly ground black pepper

INSTRUCTIONS

1. Heat the oven to 450°F. Cut
   each cabbage into 4 wedges and
   place them on a pan. Add salt
   and pepper. Pour some cream
   into the scores and top off with
   cheese.
2. Roast the cabbage in the oven
   for around 20 minutes.

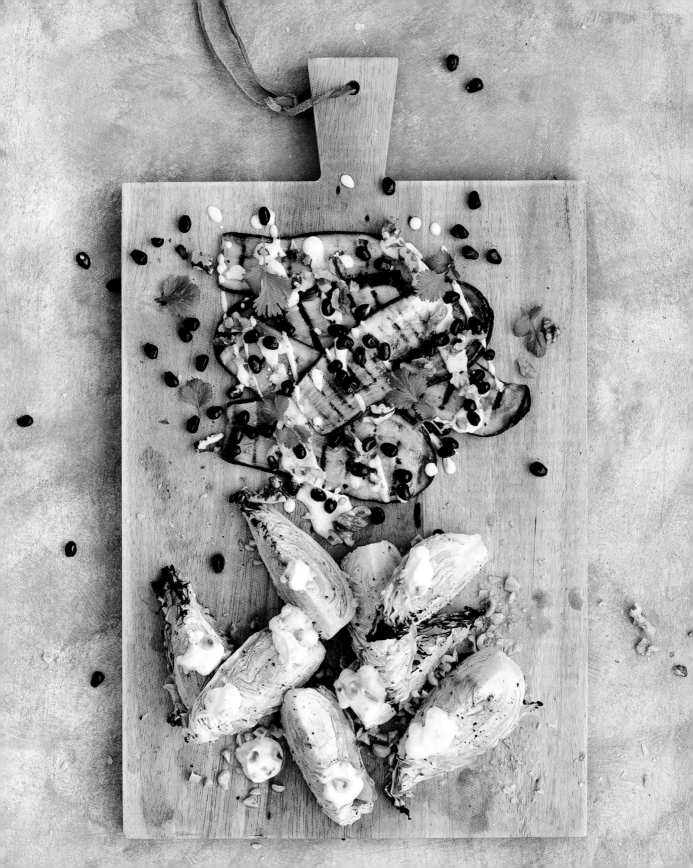

These dips are perfect for a buffet, as an appetizer, or on a piece of bread with some soup. Serve with spelt bread or gluten-free crostini.

TWO DIPS FOR THE BUFFET

Artichoke dip

2 cans artichoke hearts, just under 1 pound each (400 gram)
⅖ cup lactose-free crème fraîche
⅘ cup grated sharp cheese
Salt
Pepper
Lemon juice

INSTRUCTIONS

1. Heat the oven to 425°F. Drain the artichokes. Mix all the ingredients with a stick blender and season to taste with salt, pepper, and a dash of lemon juice.
2. Smooth a layer of the mixture, a couple of inches thick, into an oven-safe dish. Leave in the oven for 10 minutes or until the surface has turned golden.

Edamame pesto

⅖ cup edamame
3 tablespoons canola oil
A few drops concentrated garlic oil
⅕ cup pine nuts
⅘ cup grated vegetarian Parmesan
Salt
⅖ cup lactose-free crème fraîche (optional)

INSTRUCTIONS

Mix all the ingredients to make a smooth cream using a stick blender. Season to taste with salt. If you want more of a dip-like consistency, then add some crème fraîche.

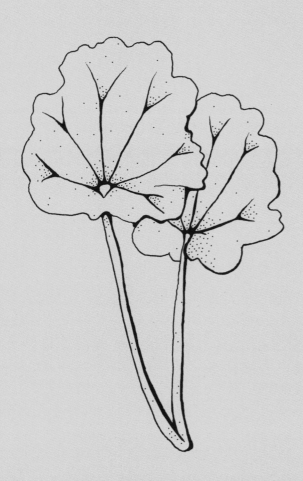

Desserts & baked goods

The world's fastest dessert. The quickest way to remove the seeds from the pomegranate is to fill a bowl with water and break up the fruit in the water. The seeds will float to the top and you avoid red splashes all over your kitchen.

ORANGE SALAD WITH POMEGRANATE

V

SERVES 4

4 oranges, a mix of normal and
    blood oranges
⅘ cup pomegranate seeds
4 tablespoons maple syrup
2 teaspoons ground cinnamon
A few fresh leaves of mint

INSTRUCTIONS

1. Remove the peel and membrane from the oranges. Cut them into slices and place on several plates or one large platter. Sprinkle over some pomegranate seeds. Drizzle the maple syrup over and dust some cinnamon on top. Garnish with fresh mint.
2. Serve the orange salad as it is or add a scoop of lactose-free vanilla ice cream.

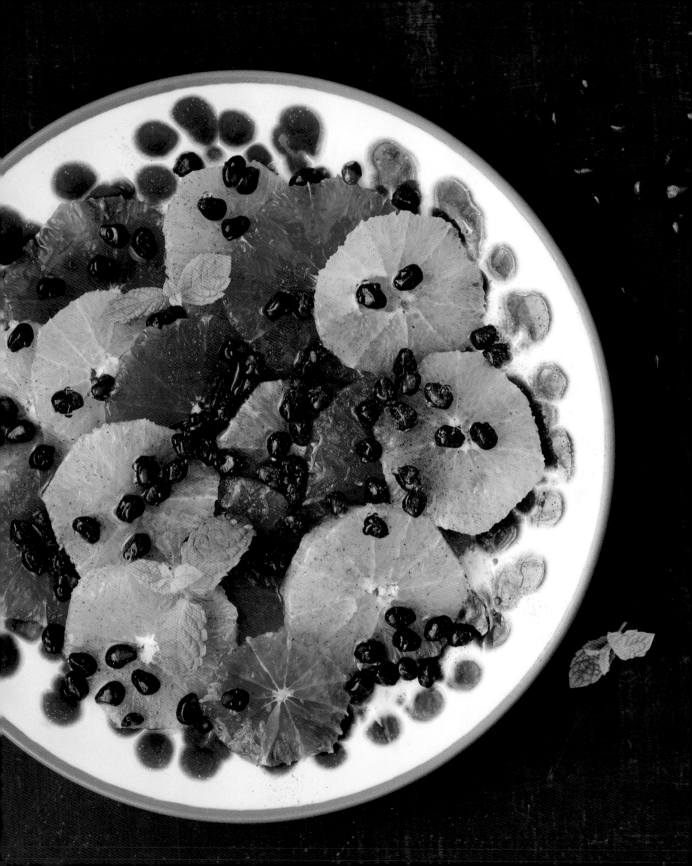

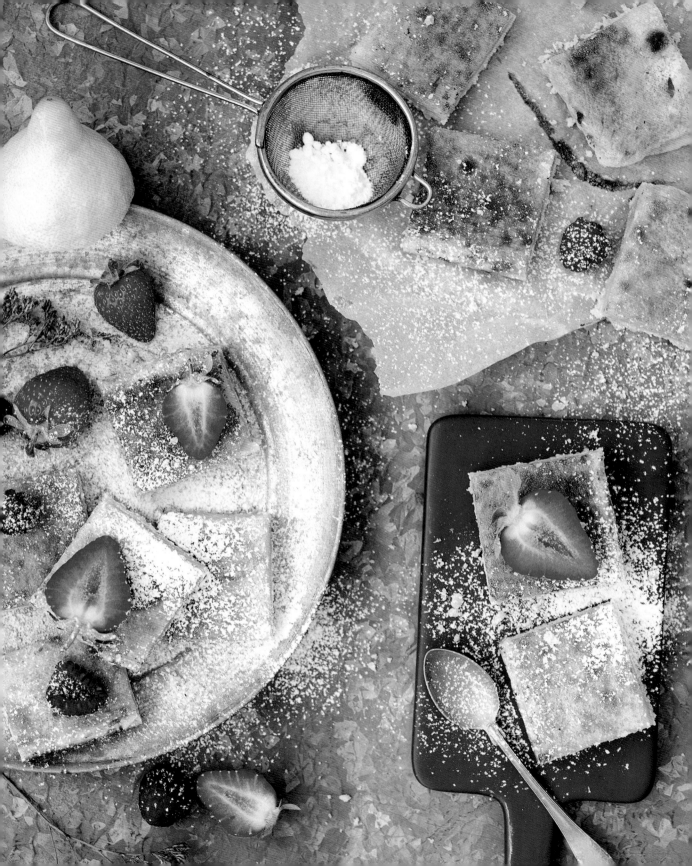

Fresh lemon-scented squares that will be eaten soon after you serve them. If you want them gluten free, you can replace the spelt flour with a gluten-free flour mixture. These squares can be frozen. Vegan? Use a dairy-free margarine and egg substitute.

LEMON SQUARES

MAKES 12

Base
1 cup sieved spelt flour
1½ tablespoons sugar
2 pinches of salt
4⅖ ounces cold butter

Filling
3 eggs
⅗ cup sugar
⅕ cup sieves spelt flour
2 teaspoons vanilla sugar
2 lemons, zest and juice
   (around ⅘ cup)

Topping
Confectioners' sugar
Fresh or frozen raspberries

INSTRUCTIONS

1. Heat the oven to 400°F. Mix the flour, sugar, and salt, and add the cold butter in pieces. Use your fingers to make a dough by pinching the butter and sugar together. Press the dough into the bottom of a springform pan lined with parchment paper (around 8 x 8 inches). Bake in the middle of the oven for around 10 minutes or until the dough starts to brown.
2. Mix eggs and sugar. Add flour, vanilla sugar, and zest and juice of the lemons. Pour the batter into the pan and bake for around 12 minutes until the cake is firm but gooey. Leave to cool and cut the cake into squares. Keep them in a cool place until ready to serve.
3. Dust with some confectioners' sugar and garnish with fresh or frozen raspberries.

A real summer dessert that works year-round. It looks fancy and tastes divine. Reduce the amount of sugar if you want the ice cream to be less sweet.

LEMON ICE CREAM IN LEMON

SERVES 4

4 lemons
⅘ cup lactose-free whipping cream
2 egg yolks
⅔ cup confectioners' sugar
3 tablespoons freshly squeezed lemon juice
⅔ cup lemon curd
⅔ cup lactose-free Greek yogurt

INSTRUCTIONS

1. Cut off the tops of the lemons and remove the flesh. Cut a little at the bottom so they can stand upright. Whisk the cream until firm. Mix the egg yolks, confectioners' sugar, lemon juice, lemon curd, and Greek yogurt in a bowl. Then carefully fold in the cream and mix.

2. Fill the lemons with the ice cream mixture. Place in the freezer for around 4 hours.

3. Remove the lemons and leave at room temperature for around 15 minutes before serving.

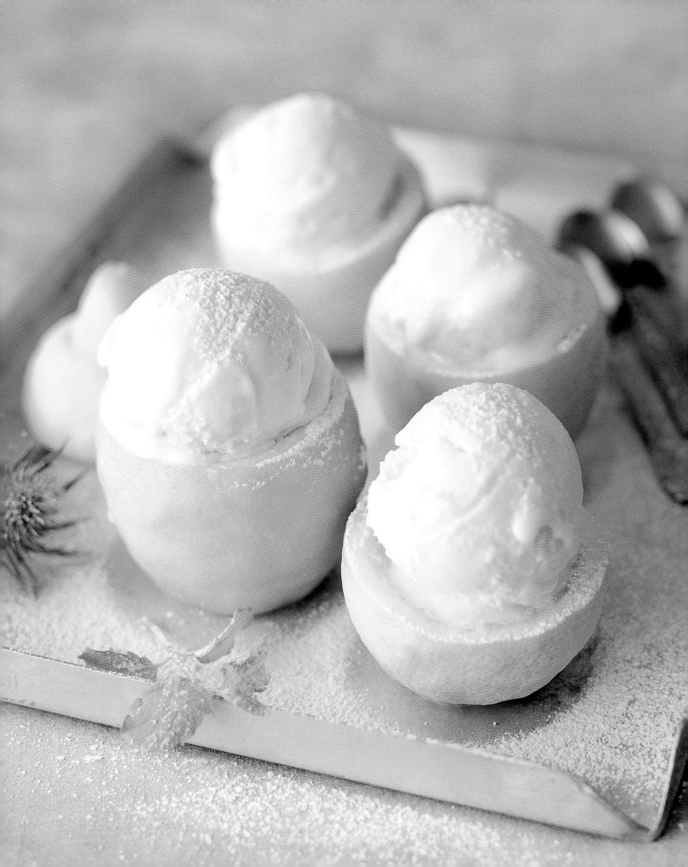

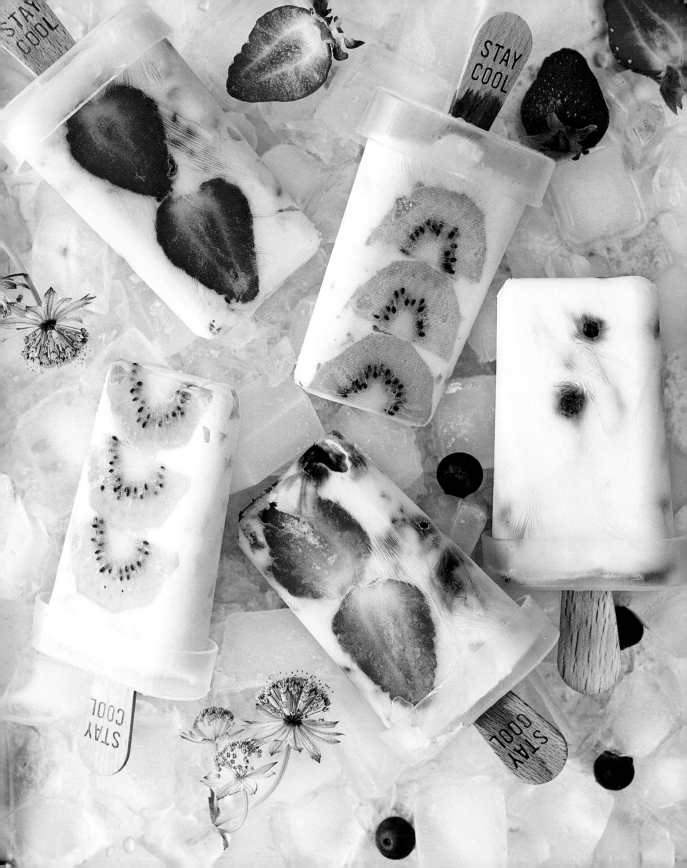

It's not always easy to find FODMAP-friendly ice cream so you might as well make it yourself. If you make double then you can freeze them and give to visitors. Vegan? Replace the Greek yogurt with oat yogurt.

FRUITY ICE CREAM LOLLIPOPS

MAKES AROUND 10

Juice of 1 lime
1⁷⁄₁₀ cup lactose-free Greek yogurt
1 teaspoon vanilla powder
1 tablespoon syrup (optional)
⅘ cup strawberries, blueberries, raspberries, and/or kiwifruit

INSTRUCTIONS

Mix the yogurt, vanilla powder, lime juice, and syrup in a bowl. Layer berries and fruit with the yogurt in Popsicle molds. Place the lollipop sticks into the molds and freeze for at least 3 hours. You can always pour some warm water on the molds to easier release the ice creams.

Toffee and pecan nuts work really well together. This pie can be addictive, but if you do have any leftovers then it will last around a week in the fridge. Vegan? Use dairy-free margarine and rice or coconut cream.

138
Desserts &
baked goods

PECAN PIE

MAKES AROUND 10 PIECES

3½ ounces butter
1¼ cup sieved spelt flour
⅓ cup granulated sugar
1 pinch salt
⅖ cup lactose-free whipping cream
⅖ cup granulated sugar
⅓ cup light syrup
2 tablespoons brown sugar
3½ ounces butter
5 ⅓ ounces pecan nuts

To serve
Lactose-free whipping cream

INSTRUCTIONS

1. Heat the oven to 400°F, Melt the butter and mix with the flour, sugar, and salt. Press the dough into a pie pan or springform pan, around 10 inches in diameter. Prick the bottom with a fork and bake in the oven for around 15 minutes.

2. Mix cream, sugar, syrup, and brown sugar in a saucepan and simmer for 10 to 15 minutes. Mix it a couple of times to stop it from burning. Add the butter and stir until everything has blended into a toffee.

3. Pour the toffee into the pecan crust. Leave to cool for a bit and then evenly sprinkle some nuts on top. Leave to cool and completely set in the fridge. Serve the pie with a lightly whipped cream.

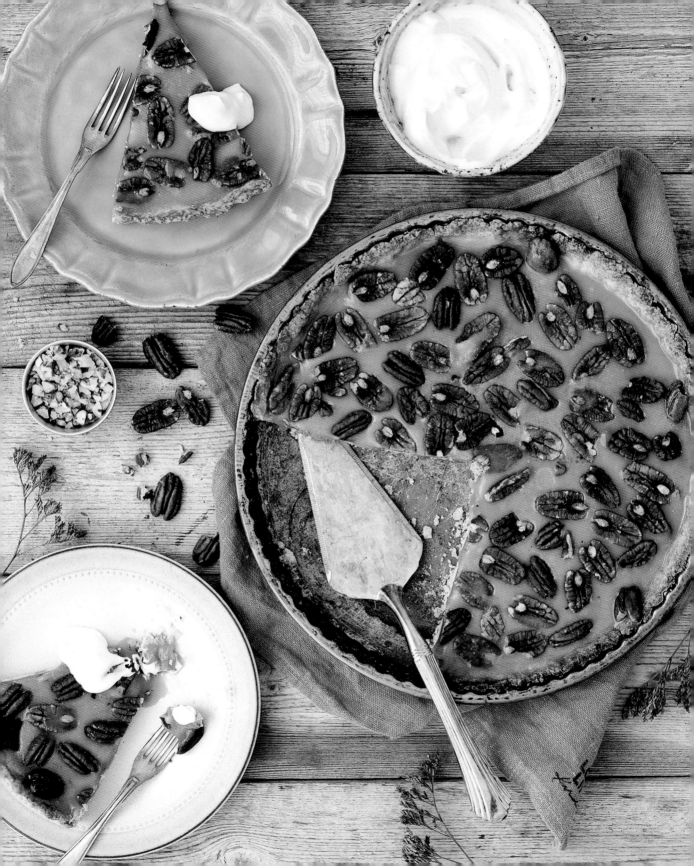

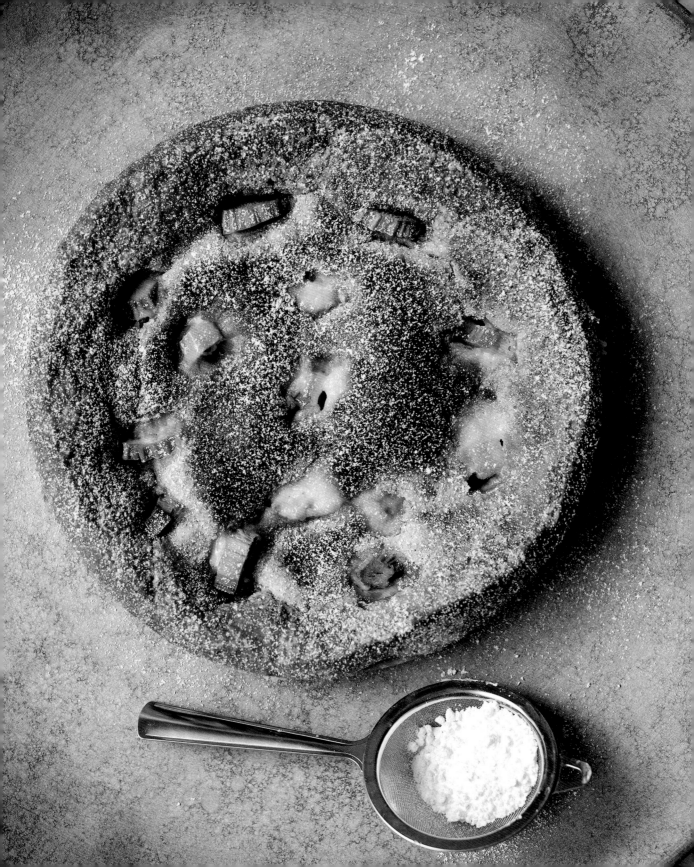

Isn't it great that rhubarb is FODMAP friendly? If you like rhubarb as much as I do, you can harvest it in the summer and freeze it. Vegan? Use dairy-free margarine, egg substitute, and dairy-free ice cream or cream.

RHUBARB CAKE

MAKES AROUND 10 PIECES

2½ ounces butter
1 teaspoon cardamom pods
2 eggs
1 cup sugar
1 teaspoon vanilla sugar
1 cup sieved spelt flour
1 teaspoon baking powder
½ pound rhubarb
2 tablespoons potato flour

To serve
Lactose-free cream or lactose-free
    vanilla ice cream

INSTRUCTIONS

1. Heat the oven to 400°F. Grease the bottom of a springform pan (or use parchment paper), around 10 inches in diameter.
2. Melt the butter and crush the cardamom pods with a mortar and pestle. Whisk the eggs, sugar, and vanilla sugar until fluffy. Mix flour and baking powder in a bowl. Mix in the flour mix, cardamom, and butter into the egg mix and pour the batter into the pan. Cut the rhubarb into ½-inch large cubes. Mix the rhubarb with the potato flour and sprinkle over the batter.
3. Bake the cake in the middle of the oven for 30 to 35 minutes. It should be slightly gooey and chewy.
4. Serve with lightly whipped cream or vanilla ice cream.

Index of recipes

Conversion charts

Metric and Imperial Conversions

(These conversions are rounded for convenience)

Ingredient	Cups/Tablespoons/ Teaspoons	Ounces	Grams/Milliliters
Butter	1 cup/ 16 tablespoons/ 2 sticks	8 ounces	230 grams
Cheese, shredded	1 cup	4 ounces	110 grams
Cream cheese	1 tablespoon	0.5 ounce	14.5 grams
Cornstarch	1 tablespoon	0.3 ounce	8 grams
Flour, all-purpose	1 cup/1 tablespoon	4.5 ounces/0.3 ounce	125 grams/8 grams
Flour, whole wheat	1 cup	4 ounces	120 grams
Fruit, dried	1 cup	4 ounces	120 grams
Fruits or veggies, chopped	1 cup	5 to 7 ounces	145 to 200 grams
Fruits or veggies, pureed	1 cup	8.5 ounces	245 grams
Honey, maple syrup, or corn syrup	1 tablespoon	0.75 ounce	20 grams
Liquids: cream, milk, water, or juice	1 cup	8 fluid ounces	240 milliliters
Oats	1 cup	5.5 ounces	150 grams
Salt	1 teaspoon	0.2 ounce	6 grams
Spices: cinnamon, cloves, ginger, or nutmeg (ground)	1 teaspoon	0.2 ounce	5 milliliters
Sugar, brown, firmly packed	1 cup	7 ounces	200 grams
Sugar, white	1 cup/1 tablespoon	7 ounces/0.5 ounce	200 grams/12.5 grams
Vanilla extract	1 teaspoon	0.2 ounce	4 grams

Oven Temperatures

Fahrenheit	Celsius	Gas Mark
225°	110°	$\frac{1}{4}$
250°	120°	$\frac{1}{2}$
275°	140°	1
300°	150°	2
325°	160°	3
350°	180°	4
375°	190°	5
400°	200°	6
425°	220°	7
450°	230°	8

Thank you!

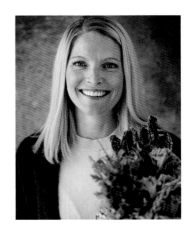

Thanks for lending me the props:
Kardelen
Mimou
R.O.O.M

Text © *Sofia Antonsson*
Photo: *Ulrika Pousette*
Design: *Anna Ågren*
Illustrations: *Surabhi Takker*
Editor: *Åsa Karsberg*
Food Director: *Madeleine Broström*
Food Stylist: *Ann-Sophie Berlin*
Props: *Anna Wendt*
Reprographics : *Italgraf Media, Stockholm*
Print: *Livonia Print*, Lettland 2018

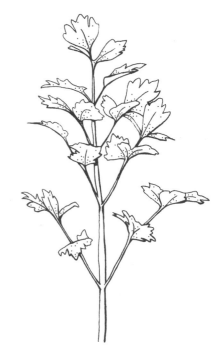

If you want to know more about IBS and
FODMAP, visit www.bellybalance.se.